SPECIFIC TECHNIQUES FOR THE PSYCHOTHERAPY OF SCHIZOPHRENIC PATIENTS

SPECIFIC TECHNIQUES FOR THE PSYCHOTHERAPY OF SCHIZOPHRENIC PATIENTS

ANDREW LOTTERMAN, M.D.
LECTURER IN PSYCHIATRY
CENTER FOR PSYCHOANALYTIC TRAINING AND RESEARCH
COLUMBIA UNIVERSITY, NEW YORK

International Universities Press, Inc.
Madison, Connecticut

INTERNATIONAL UNIVERSITIES PRESS and IUP (& design) ® are registered trademarks of International Universities Press, Inc.

Library of Congress Cataloging-in-Publication Data

Lotterman, Andrew.
   Specific techniques for the psychotherapy of schizophrenic patients / Andrew Lotterman.
      p. cm.
   Includes bibliographical references and index.
   ISBN 0-8236-6130-X (hard cover)
   1. Schizophrenia—Treatment. 2. Psychotherapy. I. Title.
   [DNLM: 1. Schizophrenia—therapy. 2. Psychotherapy—methods.
WM 203 L884s 1995]
RC514.L68 1996
616.89′820651—dc20
DNLM/DLC
for Library of Congress   95-16237
                                               CIP

Manufactured in the United States of America

Contents

Preface

I want to say a few words about the methods I used in this book to disguise case material so that patients' privacy was preserved. Scientifically, it would have been ideal if I could present case material exactly as it was, using direct quotes from therapy sessions. But, this was impossible given the need to preserve patients' anonymity. In presenting clinical illustrations, I chose to follow the method recommended by Clifft (Clifft, 1986). Clifft reviewed the recommendations of the American Psychiatric Association, the American Psychological Association and the World Psychiatric Association and developed guidelines for diguising case material. The goal is to communicate essential clinical data, while preserving the patients' anonymity. Essentially, Clifft recommends changing basic information not essential to the clinical illustration, and avoiding use of specific identifying data, and unnecessary detail. Transforming an external stressor from a death in a family to a divorce is an example of such a change in information. Similarly, a parent who has died may be described as being alive if this does not fundamentally alter the clinical sense of the material being presented. Of course, in a case where the psychodynamics revolve around a parental death, such a change should be avoided. If they do not change the essential clinical picture, false specific details may be added to disguise the patient's identity. Clifft also advocates changing specific details to more vague and general descriptions. If a patient grew up in Iowa, for example, one might describe him as being raised in the "Midwest."

In the material I present, I make no change in what one might call the "category" of a symptom. By this, I mean that if a patient has an auditory hallucination, it remains an auditory hallucination. I do not transform it into a delusion, an idea of reference, or a thought disorder. Nor do I change it into another kind of hallucination, other than auditory (e.g. tactile, or visual).

Moreover, I preserve what one might call the character of the symptom. By this I mean that if an auditory hallucination is persecutory, it remains persecutory. I do not change it into a hallucination of support or command. Within a symptom with a certain character, I may make changes in the content. For example, if a patient hears a voice telling him that his business competitors will lock him in a factory, I may disguise this by saying that the patient fears that the FBI will surround his home and prevent him from leaving.

In the clinical illustrations I discuss, I have used no direct quoted material from either patient or therapist. All of the conversations I report are paraphrased with changes made in specific words, phrases or idioms that might identify the speaker. Let us say, for example, that a patient associates a state of excited emotion with the conceptual image of "bursting" (as in "bursting with emotion"). The patient might sensationalize[1] the conceptual image of bursting in the form of feeling that his arms are expanding, and his skin is being stretched taut. In my report of this patient, I might change the conceptual image from "bursting" to "revved up," and I might report that the patient has the sensation that an engine is in his chest which is whirling around faster and faster sending vibrations throughout his body.

Making such changes in the clinical material presented a challenge. I needed to alter the account of the patient enough so that anonymity was preserved, but not so much that what was essential or particular to the original case was lost. Moreover, the patient's affect, the fantasies connected to that affect, and certain ideas or class concepts in the patient's mind, have vital links with the subsequent hallucinations, and somatic sensations. These links are crucial to understanding my ideas about deconceptualization, sensationalization, and perceptualization. While I have needed to modify quotations, and the patients' use of distinctive and identifiable words and phrases, and have also had to modify aspects of the symptom picture, I have tried to make these changes in such a way that the salience and meaning of the verbal bridges between language use and symptom formation were preserved. This process took a good deal of time and work and I

---

[1]See Chapters 4 and 6.

hope I have succeeded in preserving the sense and structure of these phenomena for the reader.

While the quotations are not exact, and some of the symptoms have been modified, I think the text presents a good overall picture of the clinical material which led me to develop my ideas about affect, thought, language, symptom formation, and psychotherapy technique in work with schizophrenic patients.

Acknowledgments

I wrote this book with a lot of help. My wife, Marcy, deserves the greatest share of credit and gratitude. She has been steady in her support and enthusiasm. During the time I spent at the library, or in my office working on this book, she always made me feel that it was time well spent. Her reading of the manuscript was fresh and insightful and her suggestions very useful. I also want to thank my daughters, Jenny and Wendy whose love and sweetness and warmth encouraged me to carry on and finally complete the book.

Dr. Ann Appelbaum spent hours reading and editing the first draft of this work. She took my ideas seriously, and made me feel that they were worth showing to others. Since the time I finished my residency, Dr. Appelbaum has helped me feel that my ideas and feelings about clinical work were worthy of attention. I am only one of many students that she has touched in this way, and I am fortunate to have had her as a teacher.

Dr. Michael Selzer supervised my work with a schizophrenic patient for a year. Dr. Selzer makes a memorable impression on all those who see him in action. In my work with him, I learned so much that was valuable and contributed to my understanding of schizophrenic patients. No symptom is too obscure or strange for Dr. Selzer to look into, and no degree of withdrawal, indifference, or negativism too daunting. Even in the most seemingly lifeless and negative patient, Dr. Selzer always looks at the slightest details of behavior and speech for signs of active will and decision making. In talking with patients, he always tries to elicit what is adult, creative, and alive. He can see flashes of irony and wry wit in the most seemingly dull and regressed behavior. He seems never to lose faith in the belief that behind the symptomatic confusion is a social and moral intelligence actively at work.

I want to thank Dr. Roberts Michels who read a later version of the manuscript and who gave a frank and fair critique. I needed someone expert in both biological psychiatry and psychoanalysis to put my ideas in perspective and to help me see my biases more clearly. I want to thank Dr. Michels for his skill and his generosity in the time he gave.

Dr. Richard Munich was very helpful in directing me in my search of the literature. His paper "Conceptual trends and issues in the psychotherapy of schizophrenia" helped orient my understanding of the history of the psychotherapy of schizophrenia and I recommend it.

Dr. Michel Quittman and Dr. Pellegrino Sarti are colleagues of mine whom I have known for years. I have learned a tremendous amount about the care of schizophrenic patients from watching these two in action, and they have taught me a great deal.

Dr. Seth Bernstein is a great friend and someone with whom I have discussed subjects large and small over the years. Like Dr. Appelbaum, he has the gift of making others feel taken seriously and his interest in my ideas enabled them to develop the courage to poke their heads into the sunlight. I want to give my warm thanks to him.

I want also to thank Dr. Richard Druss for his help over the years. A volume in itself could express only a fraction of my gratitude.

I want also to thank the therapists whose experiences and case examples helped in the development of my ideas.

Particular thanks goes to Dr. Margaret Emery, the Editor-in-Chief of International Universities Press. She has been extremely encouraging. From the outset, Dr. Emery has felt that the psychotherapy of schizophrenic patients, and the psychology of psychosis was worth teaching and learning about. I think that too little attention has been given to this subject recently, and I am very grateful to International Universities Press for recognizing its importance.

I have saved special thanks for my father. More than anyone, he encouraged me to think and to write.

For what is right and useful in this work, I want to give credit to all those whose help I have had. For what turns out to be wrong or unhelpful, I alone am responsible.

Introduction

THE ROLE OF PSYCHOLOGY

Schizophrenia is an agonizing and lonely illness. Schizophrenic patients suffer cruel emotional pain, and must bear up under tormenting feelings of humiliation, emptiness, and despair. Efforts to understand and treat schizophrenia have recruited an array of medical specialties: neurology, neurobiology, biochemistry, radiology, physiology, genetics, epidemiology, infectious disease, not to mention psychiatry, learning theory, and academic and psychodynamic psychology. The field of schizophrenia research is as fragmented as it is crowded.

We do not know what causes schizophrenia. Whenever attention shifts to one etiologic focus, whether it is anatomical, chemical, neurological, social, or psychological, each new lead disappoints our hope of finding a comprehensive cause. Each fresh discovery seems to apply only to *some* schizophrenic patients. Despite our attempts at understanding, the group of persons we call schizophrenic remains confusingly heterogeneous. Over the years, we have tried to find that singular feature of the disorder that defines what is unique and characteristic of this group: premorbid functioning, age of onset, predisposing conditions, precipitating events, symptom clusters, duration of psychosis, cognitive and social impairment, neuroanatomical and neurophysiological markers, response to biological and psychological therapies, social and work functioning, and long-term outcome. No matter how narrow the criteria for diagnosis, and how rigorously we apply them, the response to therapy and the course of these patients seem to defy reliable prediction (Hawk, Carpenter, and Strauss, 1975). We have great difficulty agreeing with one

1

another about who is schizophrenic, why they are schizophrenic, and what we as clinicians can do about it.

In this book, I will describe procedures for doing psychotherapy with schizophrenic patients. My goal is to describe a psychological therapy that is specific for schizophrenia. It is specific in that the techniques I describe are defined and delineated, and it is specific in that they address psychotherapeutic problems particular to schizophrenic patients. Because the psychological organization of schizophrenic patients differs from that of neurotic or borderline patients, I believe a distinct approach is necessary.

The heyday of psychoanalytic theories and therapies of schizophrenia extended from about 1935 to about 1975. Following this, there has been far less enthusiasm for treating schizophrenic patients with psychotherapy. Biological therapies have become the focus of attention, and, for many, the use of psychotherapy with schizophrenic patients is considered an anachronism. Some would ask why time, energy, and personnel should be wasted on a treatment that has been discredited. Why raise the hopes of patients and their families by offering a form of therapy that will only add to their frustration and disillusionment? Why pursue irrelevant psychological treatments, when there is so much evidence that the disorder has neuroanatomical, neurophysiological, neurochemical, genetic, and other biological bases?

I will respond this way: despite the understandable and deserved emphasis that has been placed on biological factors, we still have no clear understanding of the etiology of schizophrenia. Within this very diverse group of patients, each etiological factor seems to apply only to some, but not all patients, or not even to a majority of them. Impairment of the frontal lobes or ventricular enlargement is characteristic of only *some* schizophrenic individuals. A genetic pattern of inheritance seems to describe only *some* families.

Moreover, we still have only very limited success with organic treatments. It is well known that phenothiazines and like compounds do not cure schizophrenia. Usually, their effect is partial and restricted to only a segment of the schizophrenic population (Sarti and Cournos, 1990). Many schizophrenics do not respond to medication at all. For those whose "positive symptoms" (Andreason, 1985) respond, many are left with residual "negative symptoms." There is controversy about whether medication can be successfully used in treating the profoundly disabling negative symptoms at all.

On the other hand, nonpharmacological interventions do appear to help a number of patients (yet again, *some* patients, not all). Advocates of social skills training (Morrison and Bellack, 1984; Liberman, Massel, Most, and Wong, 1985; Liberman, Mueser, and Wallace, 1986) maintain that such training improves patient social functioning, and that the gains are generalized to new situations. Bellack (Bellack, Mueser, Morrison, Tierney, and Podell, 1990) report that even cognitive deficits in schizophrenia could be remediated with active training. This observation surprised the authors, who believe that the underlying deficit in schizophrenia is a lesion in the prefrontal lobes, marked by diminished blood flow.

The Vermont study (Harding, Brooks, Ashikaja, Strauss, and Breier, 1987a,b) discovered that, contrary to expectation, the majority of severely ill and chronic patients were functioning well at twenty- to twenty-five-year follow-up with 50 to 60 percent recovered or improved. These were patients whose illnesses had been severe at onset, and who had undergone frequent and long hospitalizations. They had been ill for an average of sixteen years, totally disabled for an average of ten, and continuously hospitalized for an average of six years. Many were unresponsive to an average of two-and-one-half years of phenothiazine treatment.

At the twenty to twenty-five years follow-up of patients retrospectively diagnosed as schizophrenic by DSM-III criteria (APA, 1980), 45 percent had no psychiatric symptoms. Many were leading productive, socially involved lives, and were functioning well. Of those who were still symptomatic, many managed to work around such psychotic symptoms as hallucinations and still maintain families and friends. Of those who were socially isolated, many nevertheless were able to work and support themselves.

The Vermont study shows that schizophrenia does not invariably lead to an inexorable downward course. Kraepelin's belief (1902) that schizophrenics invariably deteriorate has had a profound effect on how we think about the treatment of schizophrenia. For example, if a psychological treatment seems to help a particular patient, some would claim that the patient was not really schizophrenic. Too often, diagnosis and prognosis are collapsed into one entity. In this case, the relation between diagnosis and outcome becomes tautological. This unwarranted conceptual step has led Vaillant (1975) to emphasize that "Diagnosis and prognosis should be treated as different dimensions in psychosis."

The Vermont study suggests that schizophrenia may have many outcomes. The symptoms of some patients seem to persist stubbornly, while the symptoms and overall functioning of others appear to improve. It should be noted that at least half the patients who were studied in the Vermont research were not taking any psychotropic medication. Without discounting the important role of biological factors, the data leave room for the possibility that environmental factors may ameliorate the condition. While one can generate biological hypotheses which account for the improvements reported in the Vermont study, in fairness, one can equally well develop hypotheses based upon environmental factors. Such factors might be social, psychological, or may even involve changes in the nonhuman environment such as the effects of a pastoral setting as compared with an urban one.

We do not know where on the spectrum from the organic to the psychological, the etiological factors in schizophrenia lie. Nevertheless, whether this disorder is predominantly organic or psychological in origin, I think that psychotherapy has an important role to play.

Let us speculate that the schizophrenia is caused by a biological disturbance. Let us assume, for example, that schizophrenia is caused by a genetically determined metabolic disorder, similar to hypothyroidism. In such a case, organic factors would play an overriding causal role, and psychological influences might be irrelevant to the cause of the disorder, or even to the phenotypic expression of its symptoms. Still, successful treatment would depend on the patient's willingness to comply with his medical treatment. He must come to a clinic for periodic evaluations. He must be able to monitor the ebb and flow of his symptoms. He must be willing to take his medications regularly. No pharmacological compound can induce him to do this. No medication can lead him to accept the painful blow to his self-esteem that schizophrenia has dealt him, nor can it help him summon the courage and stamina to adapt to his disease. At the very minimum, an understanding of the psychology of schizophrenia will help us listen to and talk to such a patient. It will help us anticipate some of the patient's reactions to his illness, what forms of resistance to treatment are likely to arise, and how we might deal with these clinically.

This form of psychological work with schizophrenics has a long tradition (Sarti and Cournos, 1990). The Boston study (Stanton, Gunderson, Knapp, Frank, Vanicellia, Schnitzer, and Rosenthal, 1984; Gunderson, Frank, Katz, Vanicellia, Frosch, and Knapp, 1984) referred to it as "reality adaptive therapy." Its goal is to help the patient manage his illness as effectively as possible, to prevent relapse, and to maintain a good quality of life. Even though its goals are limited, this kind of work which schizophrenic patients is neither simple nor straightforward. Many patients must achieve considerable self-understanding in order to overcome intense denial, projection, and other distortions of reality which prevent their following through on treatment. These psychological issues are often complex, and require a lot of psychological work.

What about a model of schizophrenia in which biological factors play a less exclusive role, a model similar to that of hypertension, for example? Certainly, modern medicine believes that, for most patients, high blood pressure has a biological basis. But there is also evidence that psychological factors may play a role in the expression of symptoms. Patients have lowered blood pressure with relaxation, meditation, and other psychological techniques. What if schizophrenia is a syndrome caused by an interaction of both biological and psychological factors? This view is probably the most widely accepted one today. Carpenter (1984) has elaborated his view on the "biopsychosocial model." It is important to realize what this model actually implies. Even if there is an organic underpinning, the *expression* of the disorder, that is to say, the *type, intensity, and duration* of symptoms may depend upon environmental factors. We know of many illnesses for which an individual inherits a vulnerability, but in which the onset of frank symptoms depends upon environmental stimuli.

In these circumstances, psychological treatment may not only improve patient compliance, but may ameliorate those factors which contribute to the expression of illness. We should keep in mind that even for what appear to be biologically determined deficits such as cognitive impairment, environmental influences can, apparently, play a therapeutic role (Bellack et al., 1990). The schizophrenic patients in the Bellack study had cognitive disorders which *did* improve with active training, and these improvements endured over time. There is evidence, then, that even if elements of schizophrenia have a biological basis, environmental and psychological interventions are not wholly irrelevant.

The biopsychosocial model of schizophrenia really leaves enormous room for the role of psychotherapy. At one theoretical extreme, we can imagine that biological lesions directly dictate the expression of overt symptoms. As I mentioned above, psychotherapy can then help the patient manage his disease, or, more ambitiously, as in the case of the patients with cognitive deficits, to treat the expression of the disorder. It is entirely possible, however, that biological factors do not penetrate directly to symptom expression, but act through intermediate levels of function. Some of these levels may be more physiological, and some more psychological in nature. For example, schizophrenia may involve a disorder of stimulus thresholds, which impinge on the psychological apparatus in various ways. Social isolation and flattened affect may be attempts by the patient to shield himself from trauatic levels of stimulation. Or, schizophrenic patients may have greater inborn levels of aggression or vulnerability to frustration which then call upon such defenses as anergy, avolition, or the disorganization of behavior. Or, the biological disturbance may affect a more obviously psychological level of function. For example, there may be constitutional differences in ego functioning (e.g., the capacity for delay, synthesis, or symbol use) which directly or indirectly affects behavior and which also calls various psychological defenses into play.

The notion that psychological factors can have a material impact on biological processes should not be dismissed as fanciful or unscientific. Jensen, Bnefke, Hyldebrandt, Pedersen, Petersen, and Weile (1982) reported cerebral atrophy in torture victims. Recent animal studies demonstrate that, in species as primitive as fish, social experience in the external world produces biochemical changes in the internal world. Davis and Fernald (1990), Fernald, (1993) report that African cichlid fish (*Haplochronis burtoni*) respond to *perceived* (by the fish) changes in their social environment with changes in brain tissue. When brightly colored, dominant male fish lose a territorial battle with a rival, they shrink in size and lose their coloration. Moreover, GnRH-secreting neurons[1] in the preopticohypothalamic complex shrink in size. These anatomical and physiological changes, which are reliably measurable, result not from any anatomical lesion, but from what one might call a social, or to be precise, a mental lesion. After their losing effort, the cichlid fish perceive themselves as occupying a different status in their social order. Physical changes do not precede, but rather follow that perception. Davis and Fernald write, "It remains to be understood just how a change in an individual male's *perception* of his social status is translated into increased cell growth and GnRH production " (p. 1187). I do not think it unscientific to hypothesize that these fish have an inner realm which could be termed *mental*. It is not the array of visual images which flashes across their retina, or the sounds which activate auditory neurons that are unique here. After all, victorious fish will experience roughly similar physical sensations. Rather, it is the meaning or significance of these sensations that is assigned to them by the fish that is decisive; the fact that they have *won* rather than *lost* the battle for dominance. This suggests, I think, that there is some kind of experiential realm, even in fish, which is involved in registering "meanings" no matter how rudimentary or primitive. If this is so, even in discussing fish, perhaps we might consider the concept of "mind" and distinguish it from "brain." Evidence suggests that this "mind," this realm of "significance," has its own material impact on brain and biochemistry.

Research on obsessive–compulsive disorder in humans also suggests that changes in the external environment can produce anatomical and physiological changes in the internal biochemical milieu. Neziroglu, Steele, Yaryura-Tobias, Hitri, and Diamond (1990) reported changes in the levels of serotonin metabolites in the brains of patients with obsessive–compulsive disorder. Before behavior therapy these levels were elevated compared to normal controls. After behavior therapy, metabolite levels returned to normal. These levels were similar to those in patients who had been successfully treated with fluoxetine and chlorimipramine.

---

[1]These neurons secrete growth hormone releasing hormone.

Baxter et al. (Baxter, Schwartz, Bergman, Szuba, Guze, Mazziota, Alazraki, Selin, Ferng, Munford, and Phelps, 1992) have reported that cerebral metabolic rates for glucose in patients with obsessive–compulsive disorder were lowered both by fluoxetine hydrochloride treatment and by behavior therapy. Again, this is evidence that mental and behavioral events can change brain biochemistry.

However complicated the interplay of environment and neurophysiology may be, these studies suggest that thoughts and behavior can have a material impact on neurophysiology. To put it another way, just as molecules can move mind, mind can move molecules. The current doctrine that mind is to be reduced to brain may result as much from the current bias of the scientific community as from fact. Neither science nor logic can fairly justify the reduction of mind to brain. This is important, I think, because there is a bias within the scientific culture (to some extent, including psychiatry) that psychological elements are not "real," and that they are essentially epiphenomena of biochemistry. What commerce there is between the two is considered a one-way street in which biology determines thought, and not vice versa. The view that elements of mind have legitimate scientific status in their own right, and should be studied as such, is sometimes thought to be antiquated and scientifically soft headed.

Be this as it may, these studies do support the idea that brain and mind are intimately connected. Whatever the level at which functioning is disrupted in schizophrenia, whether closer to the level of brain or closer to the level of mind, the biopsychosocial model leaves open the possibility that psychological intervention can play a role in reducing symptoms.

Finally, of course, there is the possibility that psychological factors, at least for some patients diagnosed as schizophrenic, may play a causal role (see the cases of the two patients with "hysterical psychosis" described in chapter 1). It should be kept in mind that psychoanalytic psychology is a very young discipline. The study of the ego and its functioning, and of the disruptions of that functioning, is younger still. The psychology of severely pathological mental states is not easy to grasp for people who are successfully adapted to the common culture. Usual forms of empathy and understanding often fail when we try to understand the mental experience of patients whose thought processes are so different from our own. For most of this century the mainstream of psychoanalysis has focused on the psychology of neurotics. When that psychology was applied to more severe conditions such as borderline personality disorder, it was not especially effective (Kernberg, 1975). Only when less familiar forms of psychological functioning were identified, for example, the defenses of splitting, primitive denial, and projective identification, was progress made in the treatment of these conditions.

I believe that something similar may have happened in the case of schizophrenia. It is very hard to empathize with the experience of a deluded, hallucinated, or thought disordered schizophrenic patient. The psychological mechanisms in schizophrenia are likely to differ quite markedly from those of neurotic patients and from those of normal or neurotic researchers and clinicians. Many psychological processes germane to the causes of schizophrenia, and to its treatment, may not yet have been identified. If this is so, and I believe that it is, then further psychological study of schizophrenia has value and meaning.

PSYCHOTHERAPY AS A TREATMENT

Research about the effectiveness of psychotherapy is a new area of study. It has just begun to define its subject matter and to develop its methods. When this is combined with the fact that human behavior and mental functioning are breathtakingly complex, we must be cautious about interpreting the results of current psychotherapy research. Nevertheless, there are some studies which suggest that the psychotherapy of schizophrenic patients may have a beneficial effect. A number of early outcome studies were inconclusive and suffered from methodological problems. However, a more recent investigation, the Boston study (Stanton et al., 1984; Gunderson et al., 1984) showed that expressive, insight-oriented psychotherapy had a beneficial effect on schizophrenic patients, and that this differed from the effect of supportive or reality adaptive therapy. The exploratory therapy that was studied consisted of a rather traditional insight-oriented approach that focused on intensive interaction three times per week, understanding of motivation and transference phenomena, the development of insight, the interpretation of the symbolic meaning of symptoms, self-observation, and the use of clarification and interpretation. The reality adaptive therapy was nonintensive and focused on current complaints. In this form of treatment, the therapist used a combination of support, reassurance, and direction. The exploratory therapy seemed to produce improvements in ego functioning, while the reality therapy improved the patient's occupational and social functioning.

A later study (Glass, Katz, Schnitzer, Knapp, Frank, and Gunderson, 1989) found that the more expert a therapist was at exploratory therapy, the better the outcome. Better technique was associated with decreased levels of denial, diminished apathy, and a decrease in retarded functioning.

While the Boston study has its own methodological problems, it has the virtue of demonstrating that psychotherapy can be associated with a reduction of symptoms in schizophrenics, that different techniques have differential effects, and that more successful applications of technique are associated with better outcomes.

Another recent study (Frank and Gunderson, 1990) reported that a positive therapeutic alliance with schizophrenic patients was associated with greater participation in therapy, increased compliance with medication, better overall functioning, and less use of medication.

These studies show that environmental influences, and in particular psychotherapy, may have an impact on the course of schizophrenia. Given the current emphasis in psychiatry on the role of biology, this bears attention. Certainly, further studies will be helpful.

These studies do not address a very important question, however: What specific procedures does one use to do psychotherapy with a schizophrenic patient? Does one conduct unmodified psychodynamic psychotherapy? Should one modify traditional psychodynamic or psychoanalytic technique to address the specific combination of deficits and conflicts that these patients present? Many authors have noted that it is very hard for schizophrenic patients to form a therapeutic alliance (Freud, 1937; Fenichel, 1945; Fromm-Reichmann, 1959; Carpenter, 1984; Frank and Gunderson, 1990). The relationships that these patients develop are often very intense, but very brittle. How does one interact with the patient to address this special problem? Schizophrenic patients may have profound disturbances of thought and speech.

How does one conduct a psychotherapy whose main tools are concepts and words, if a patient has a thought disorder such as looseness of association? Schizophrenic patients can be suddenly, impulsively, and primitively aggressive. Does one conduct traditional, unmodified exploratory psychotherapy with such patients? If so, when the patient tries to untie your shoe or burn your jacket, what do you do? The images these patients have of themselves and of others is often very distorted. They can behave as if the boundaries between themselves and others have evaporated. A patient may take coins from your desk or books from your shelf. How does one conceptualize these behaviors, and how does one address them in psychotherapy?

The psychotherapy studies cited above do not address these issues. In some ways, this is understandable since the technology of psychotherapy research in general, and of the research concerning the psychotherapy of schizophrenic patients in particular, is so new and at such a formative stage. Even the classic anecdotal literature written by well-known clinicians, however, has neglected to specify particular techniques and link them with specific symptoms. Often, these writers have focused on the dynamic etiology or metapsychology of schizophrenia (Freud, 1911, 1923, 1924a, b; Hartmann, 1949, 1953; Jacobson, 1964). When technique has been discussed, it has been in a rather amorphous way (Fromm-Reichmann, 1959).

In order to put this book in context, I would like to review the psychoanalytic concept of structural diagnosis (see also chapter 1). Commonly in psychiatry, as in medicine, diagnosis is descriptive: various symptoms and signs of a disorder are collected together and identified as a syndrome. When a specific etiological factor is found, a disease is identified (Andreason, 1985). In medicine in general, diagnoses are used to guide treatment decisions. Patients with syndrome A are found to respond to treatment X. This is equally true in psychiatry. For example, DSM-III-R (APA, 1987) has defined psychiatric syndromes for which various treatments are prescribed. In psychiatry, as in medicine, such syndromes are often treated with organic remedies; these include pharmacotherapy, electroconvulsive therapy (ECT), and light therapy.

The relationship between diagnosis and psychological treatment has been much less clear. Until relatively recently, psychiatric diagnosis had little to do with psychotherapy and how it is conducted. The psychodynamic therapist simply focused on dynamic themes and used clarification, confrontation, and interpretation as his tools. Whether a patient was hysterical, obsessive, psychopathic, inhibited, impulsive, or psychotic made relatively little difference. In general, diagnosis, as it related to psychotherapy practice, played a very minor role. (When a clinician thought a patient was not amenable to insight work, the patient was treated with supportive and manipulative techniques.)

Eissler (1953a) was one of the first to provide a conceptual framework for modifying psychoanalytic technique according to the patient's particular psychology. He emphasized that one might have to modify traditional technique based upon the presence of certain pathological modifications of the patient's ego. If the psychological disorder had impaired the patient's ego functioning, the patient would not be able to participate in a "basic model" of psychoanalysis. Eissler suggested, in fact, that one might make a diagnosis of the patient's ego functioning based on the extent to which he could participate in a "basic model" psychoanalysis.

Kernberg (1975, 1984; Kernberg, Selzer, Koenigsberg, Carr, and Appelbaum, 1989) followed in Eissler's path, and developed a diagnostic system that was not only descriptive, but also structural. Whereas descriptive diagnosis had only guided clinicians in selecting organic forms of treatment, the structural diagnosis might guide clinicians in the application of psychological methods of treatment. For Kernberg, the use of traditional psychoanalytic therapy was not appropriate for certain patients with severe character disorders. Such patients were impulsive, expressed excessive amounts of unmodified aggression, and devalued their therapists. Moreover, they acted self-destructively in ways that overwhelmed traditional verbal therapies. Also, their use of primitive defenses made it impossible for more traditional forms of transference neurosis to develop, but produced instead grossly distorted transferences which often had little to do with actual early experience. These patients' behavior frequently made it impossible for the therapist to remain neutral, and able to think calmly about the clinical material. Based on his view of the specific causes of ego weakness in these patients, Kernberg proposed modifications of traditional technique. These modifications included the use of limit setting; structuring the treatment in the initial phase so as to reduce acting out and self-destructiveness; a focus on the interpretation of the transference in the here-and-now; a focus on the confrontation and interpretation of such primitive defenses as splitting and projective identification; and a focus on the confrontation and interpretation of negative transference. These techniques were intended to address the specific psychotherapeutic problems of a specific patient group—borderline patients. These changes in technique were intended to deal with symptoms that sprang from a particular psychological structure which differed from that of the neurotic patient. The goal of these modifications was to increase the power and specificity of psychotherapy with this particular patient group.

Clearly, schizophrenic patients are very different from the kinds of neurotic patients for whom psychoanalytic therapy was first invented. Nevertheless, there has been little written about how traditional technique should be specifically modified to treat these patients. Most of what has been written from a psychoanalytic viewpoint, has focused on questions of etiology. Those accounts which have examined technical issues have often been nonspecific and vague. Some authors have provided extremely provocative and stimulating reports of their work and clinical theory (Bion, 1957; Searles, 1962, 1979) but have not tried to systematize their recommendations about therapy. Several authors (Semrad, Menaer, Mann, and Standish, 1952; Will, 1975) have given some very useful general guidelines (e.g., "Stop, look and listen"), but omit details about how to address specific clinical problems in working with schizophrenic patients. They do not tell us how, for example, to approach thought disorder, looseness of association, provocative behavior, delusions, or countertransference disgust and rage. Moreover, these writers do not link their recommendations with a specific formulation about how schizophrenic patients differ structurally from neurotic or borderline patients.

Federn (1934, 1943a,b,c) is a notable exception. He did present a set of recommendations for psychotherapy with schizophrenic patients based upon his views of the specific defects in their ego functioning. He developed his technical prescriptions deliberately out of his clinical theory. While I do not agree with many of his conclusions about the psychology of schizophrenia or its treatment, he deserves credit for attempting to link a structural diagnosis with psychotherapy technique.

My aim in this book is to identify and describe psychological mechanisms which may be at work in schizophrenia. I will describe a treatment approach which tries to take into account the fact that the psychology of schizophrenia is different from the psychology of neurosis or borderline conditions. I present these views not in order to discount the amassed evidence that biological processes are implicated in the symptoms of many schizophrenic patients, but rather to broaden and deepen a complimentary, not an antagonistic, psychological point of view.

Before I close this introduction, I would like to say a word about methodology. The data I will present are clinical and anecdotal, like most psychoanalytic reports. It is based on work with twenty or so patients over the course of about fifteen years. The sample is small, and the data are not derived from a statistically sophisticated research design. I cannot "certify" that the observations I have made apply to all patients, or that the phenomena I describe cannot be explained in ways other than mine. But despite the absence of a controlled design and statistical corroboration, I think this kind of clinical research is worthwhile. Before systematic research can occur, hypotheses need to be generated and explored clinically. My aim is to present the work I have done, to describe my clinical findings, and to offer them for the reader's consideration.

Chapter 1

Diagnosis and Patient Sample

The most important use of diagnosis in medicine is to make treatment decisions. The purpose of history taking, physical examination, gram stains, bacterial cultures, X rays, and so on, in a patient with fever and a productive cough, is to direct the physician to one form of treatment rather than another. His diagnostic impression may lead him to prescribe antibiotics rather than a diuretic, for example.

Diagnosis plays the same role in psychiatric treatments. Both from a biological and psychological standpoint, diagnosis should, ideally, help guide practice. Because of this, and because it is important to describe how the patients discussed in this book were identified as schizophrenic, I would like to review the issue of diagnosis.

Controversy has surrounded the descriptive diagnosis of schizophrenia since the time of Kraepelin. Most authors agree that the term *schizophrenia* denotes an extremely heterogeneous group of conditions in which symptoms may be mild or severe, remitting or chronic, early or relatively late occurring, quietly devastating or floridly dramatic. The term has experienced a considerable evolution in descriptive psychiatry.

Modern descriptive diagnosis began with Kraepelin (1902)[1] who developed the concept of "dementia praecox" to distinguish the disorder from manic-depressive illness. He believed that the illness had an early onset and progressed inexorably on a downhill course to dementia. Symptoms included hallucinations, delusions, withdrawal, poor judgment, difficulty with concentration

---

[1]Much of this section on descriptive diagnosis draws upon *The Treatment of Acute Psychotic Episodes* (Levy and Ninan, 1990).

and attention, and disconnection between ideas and affect. Kraepelin's diagnosis relied heavily on the course or outcome of the disease: if a patient did not have a deteriorating course, most likely he did not have schizophrenia.

Eugen Bleuler (1911) characterized schizophrenics not by their course, but by their cross-sectional symptoms. His "fundamental" symptoms included: association, affect (disturbed), autism, and ambivalence. Hallucinations and delusions were thought to arise secondarily from the fundamental symptoms.

Schneider (1959) also rejected the idea of defining schizophrenia by its course. He developed another list of cross-sectional symptoms that he termed *first rank*. These included such phenomena as auditory hallucinations in which voices comment on one's actions or argue, thought withdrawal, thought insertion, and delusions of control or passivity. In an effort to define this group of patients, Carpenter, Strauss, and Bartko (1973) developed another symptom list which included restricted affect, incoherent speech, nihilism, and delusions.

The problem with many of the cross-sectional approaches was their lack of specificity and poor correlation with outcome.

Feighner, Robins, Guze, Woodruff, Winokur, and Munoz (1972) combined a list of cross-sectional symptoms with a time span for duration and onset. What was called The Research Diagnostic Criteria drew from Feighner and Schneider's work and ultimately became the basis for diagnosing schizophrenia in DSM-III and DSM-III-R (APA, 1980, 1987). The presence of some combination of delusions, hallucinations, thought disorder, flat or inappropriate affect, and deteriorated work or social functioning define the illness. There is a six-month duration criterion for inclusion. Thus, the course of the disorder is included along with cross-sectional symptoms in developing the diagnosis.

DSM-III-R recognized "spectrum" features to schizophrenia. Those who have the disorder for less than six months are labeled *schizophreniform,* and those who do not quite meet the full diagnostic criteria are termed *schizotypal.* Research proceeds in determining the reliability and validity of these diagnostic entities. One trouble with diagnostic criteria that include course is that they are tautological. Ninan (1990) writes, "However, when the course of illness itself is part of the diagnostic criteria (i.e., symptoms present for at least six months in the DSM-III-R criteria) such arguments become inherently circular in nature, and are of limited value" (p. 2). This becomes important in evaluating psychotherapy technique and outcome. If one finds that schizophrenic symptoms seem to improve with psychotherapy, one may be faced with the objection that the patient was, after all, not schizophrenic. Even if such a patient meets all cross-sectional criteria, as well as the criterion of six-month duration, the traditional association between downhill course and diagnosis is strong in the minds of many. That such a patient could improve with psychotherapy meets with considerable skepticism.

The purpose of DSM-III and DSM-III-R has been to operationalize terms, to classify overt and objectifiable behavior so as to develop valid and reliable criteria for research use. This promises to reduce a great deal of confusion in research and treatment efforts.

However, these diagnostic systems do not address what goes on in the minds of schizophrenic patients, and therefore tell us little about how to modify psychotherapy technique. For example, they do not differentiate between a formerly "schizophrenic" patient who no longer meets DSM-III-R criteria and a patient with character pathology. Yet, the psychological functioning of the once overtly schizophrenic patient may be very different from the patient with personality disorder. Defenses may be more primitive, fantasies more distorted, selfobject boundaries more porous, emotional life more empty, symbol use more disturbed, relatedness more fragile, and the more subtle aspects of reality testing more compromised. To make these distinctions, which are more relevant in guiding psychotherapy practice, one needs to make a psychodynamic diagnosis.

With some exceptions (Kernberg, 1970), psychoanalysis, the driving force behind most psychodynamic psychotherapy, has not been systematic in classifying the patients it treats. The same may be said of those who have worked with schizophrenic patients in psychotherapy. A number of early workers in this area (Fromm-Reichmann, 1959; Sullivan, 1962; Searles, 1962; Bion, 1957) did not concern themselves much with diagnostic issues. These authors provided clinical descriptions of symptoms such as hallucinations, delusions, social anxiety, and withdrawal, and in some cases descriptions of differences in defensive functioning (Bion, 1957; Searles, 1962, 1979). But they did not delineate how the mental structures of these patients differ from those of neurotics or borderline patients. As a result, it is difficult at times to tell whether the patients they talk about are borderline, schizotypal, schizophreniform, schizophrenic, bipolar, or hysterical.

The differences between schizophrenics and neurotics seem for some writers to be quantitative: schizophrenics have more intense symptoms that arise from more intense conflict, and are generated at earlier stages of development. These writers believe that while dynamic conflict in schizophrenia is more intense, it occurs on a continuum with the normal. For some writers, the dynamic conflicts themselves are believed to be simply more intense versions of those we recognize in neurotic patients, albeit elaborated in a "schizophrenic" way.

Nevertheless, these authors have made some intriguing points concerning diagnosis. Bion (1957) emphasized that schizophrenics, despite their psychosis, maintain areas of their personality which are nonpsychotic and which must be addressed. Katan (1954) made a similar point.

Searles (1979) maintains that certain countertransference reactions are a reliable guide in telling him if he is dealing with a schizophrenic patient. He writes:

> One of the surest criteria I have discovered, by which to know that a patient is schizophrenic, is my finding that I tend to experience myself as being nonhuman in relation to him—to feel, for example, that I emerge, in relation to him, as being so inhumanly callous or sadistic, or so filled with weird fantasies within myself, as to place me well outside the realms of human beings. . . . The one main point which I wish to make here is to caution against our taking refuge, collectively, in an orientation toward our patients . . . an orientation in which we tend to think of psychotic patients primarily in terms of objectifying them for diagnostic purposes—trying to discern wherein they differ from their fellow men, including, of course, ourselves—and in which we attempt to select this or that drug with the hoped-for magical power to reach the patient and affect his thinking and his feeling, without our own selves, our own feelings and private thinking, becoming much involved [p. 285].

Schizophrenic patients in Searles' view profoundly resist adopting a defined, circumscribed identity because they seek to avoid a kind of spiritual death. They fear that any one identity will be too constricting and impoverishing.

Many psychoanalytic writers have tried to formulate more formal criteria for psychosis.[2] Freud (1924a,b) understood the heart of psychosis to be the rupture in the relation of the ego to the external world. By means of disavowal, the ego denies intolerable external frustrations, and if need be, tolerates a disruption in its own unity (i.e., splitting). Disavowal leads psychotic patients to experience a "loss of reality."

In accounting for symptoms of psychosis, analytic writers have proceeded down two related paths: (1) examining the nature of the patients' relationship to reality, and (2) examining the boundary between the self and the object.

Weissman (1958) delineated the difference between *reality sense* and *reality testing*. Reality sense refers to the feeling or emotional conviction that attaches to a perception, which may be separate from the intellectual acceptance of its existence. Reality testing refers to processes such as perception, the recognition of enduring changes in an external object caused by action taken upon it, and the observation of predictable and repeatable transformations in objects that one uses to determine whether a phenomenon exists in the external world. Weissman also touched on something developed by Kernberg later—the social component or reality testing, or the "corroborative element." While what is real is not a matter for popular vote, nevertheless, the capacity of the individual to appreciate social norms and to determine the presence or absence of the corroboration of others, is important. To give an example: a 45-year-old schizophrenic woman attended the clinic during both summer and winter wearing several layers of sweaters. When I asked about this, she seemed very surprised that I thought it worthy of discussion and seemed puzzled that I found it unusual. She could not empathize with my puzzlement.

Frosch (1964) in his paper "The Psychotic Character" also distinguished between the *feeling of reality* (equivalent to Weissman's *sense of reality*) and *reality testing*. Frosch also described what

---

[2]The terms *psychosis* and *schizophrenia* will be used interchangeably here. The psychology of affective disorders is not a focus of this work.

he termed the *relationship to reality*, that is, the "capacity to perceive the external and internal world and the appropriateness of [the patient's] relationship to them" (p. 84). A satisfactory relationship to reality presupposes the capacity to distinguish between self and other. A schizophrenic patient had holed up in her apartment, letting bills pile up, provoking eviction notices, and threats to cut off hot water and electricity. Out of concern, her neighbor acted as a kind of auxiliary ego. When the patient was asked about her disregard for her precarious condition, she remained utterly indifferent, and, indeed, was even annoyed that the psychiatrist had intruded on her personal business. Her relationship to reality was disturbed.

The theme of confusion between self and object has been addressed by many psychoanalytic authors (Freud, 1930, pp. 57–146; Winnicott, 1953; Jacobson, 1954, 1964, 1967; Little, 1958; Mahler, 1968; Stoller, 1974; Loewald, 1980). Freud (1930) wrote, "An infant at the breast does not as yet distinguish his ego from the external world" (pp. 66–67). He goes on to say, "Originally the ego includes everything, later it separates off an external world from itself" (p. 68). For Freud, in early development and in psychopathology the "boundaries of the ego" differ from those of the normal adult.

Fenichel (1945) referred to the "indistinct ego boundaries" (p. 423) in schizophrenia, the "merging of the cathexes of object representations and of the ego" (p. 420), and to the ego's lack of differentiation from the outside world.

Jacobson (1954, 1957, 1964, 1967) focused on the development of self and object images. For her, schizophrenics suffer from a breakdown in the boundaries between self and object representations. This breakdown permits the upsurge of "drive diffusion, and drive deneutralization and (leads) to a flooding of the ego with sexual and especially with destructive and self-destructive forces to the point of a regressive dissolution of psychic structures" (1967, p. 47). For Jacobson, not only is there a refusion of self and object images in schizophrenia, but also an unleashing of primitive aggression and a dissolution of the ego and superego as distinct structures.

Mahler (1968) also maintained that fusion of self and object images and dedifferentiation are implicated in psychosis. Many other psychoanalytic writers have echoed these themes.

More recently, Kernberg (1975, 1984) has combined the emphasis on defects in reality testing and self-object differentiation in his "structural" diagnosis of psychosis. He defines reality testing as the capacity to differentiate intrapsychic from external origins of perception, self from nonself, and the capacity to realistically evaluate one's own behavior, affect, and thought in terms of ordinary social norms (Kernberg, 1984, p. 18). The capacity to empathize with the social criteria of reality is the most sensitive marker of psychotic structure, and may be impaired even in the absence of perceptual problems or lack of self-object differentiation. In Kernberg's structural interview (1984, pp. 27–51), confrontation of inappropriate behavior, thought, or affect and confrontation or interpretation of primitive defenses help differentiate schizophrenic from borderline patients. According to Kernberg, schizophrenic patients will regress and show deterioration of functioning following such interventions. In paranoid patients, this method may run into difficulty. Paranoid patients are often guarded and maintain islands of intact ego function, and so, may successfully evade disclosure of psychotic thought processes. It may take several interviews to distinguish between paranoid psychosis and paranoid character (Kernberg, 1984, p. 46).

Several writers have tried to identify psychotic patients by means of the characteristic nature of their defenses. Freud (1923, 1924a,b) described the use of disavowal in psychotic patients. He believed that disavowal contributed to the disturbance in the relation to reality which was the hallmark of the disorder.

Jacobson (1957) picked up this theme and discussed the relationship between denial and psychosis. For Jacobson, denial may be used against either external or internal phenomena. Denial leads to segregating off, or splitting off areas of affect or cognition. Unlike repression, it is not selective and compels the ego far more to compromise its unity. It is a primitive, massive, and nonselective effort to defend against instinct, ideas, and perceptions. In repression, the ego responds to signal anxiety by erecting a barrier against selected impulses, affects, and ideas. In denial, the ego acts as if the danger signal were not there, as if the threatening impulses, affects, and ideas did not exist. Thus there can be a denial of internal reality as well as external perception. What Hartmann has termed *internal reality testing* is disrupted (1953, pp. 200–202). Denial is therefore implicated in a disturbed relation to both external and internal reality, and to a massive compromise of the unity of the ego.

As has been noted, Jacobson suggested that the refusion of self and object images is a defensive operation which leads to compromised reality testing and psychosis. Also implicated are the use of primitive introjective and projective mechanisms based on early forms of identification.

Mahler (1968) also described the operation of primitive ego mechanisms ("maintenance mechanisms") in psychosis. These include dedifferentiation, deanimation, devitalization, and fusion and refusion of self and object images.

Finally, Kernberg (1975, 1984) also describes the operation of primitive defenses such as splitting, projective identification, and refusion of self and object images in the psychology of psychosis. These operations, which are used to reduce conflict and anxiety, eventually victimize the ego to such a degree that reality testing is compromised.

The various viewpoints described here demonstrate that diagnosing schizophrenia is not a well-defined procedure. Descriptive diagnoses have the advantage of being operational and well defined, but they often lack specificity, and in view of their reliance on course, are, to some degree, circular. Psychoanalytic diagnoses address the issue of subjective experience, the organization of the mind, ego functioning, and defensive operations which are relevant to psychotherapy technique. However, they are often imprecise and subjective, lacking interobserver reliability. In chapter 3, I will present my own view of psychic structure in schizophrenia. I will leave that discussion for the later chapter because I want to emphasize the link between structural diagnosis and technique. In addition, at that point, the reader will have become sufficiently familiar with the patient sample that I can draw upon them for case illustrations.

In selecting patients to discuss in this book, I have used both DSM-III-R and Kernberg's classification in evaluating patients described here. All the patients meet DSM-III-R criteria for schizophrenia except one, Mr. Tilden. This patient clearly meets criteria for schizotypal disorder, but it is a matter of viewpoint as to whether he meets criteria for schizophrenia (i.e., whether he fulfills four out of seven, or five out of seven of the necessary criteria;

see DSM-III-R [1987, pp. 187–198]). I include him in the discussion because even though he may not fulfill DSM-III-R criteria, I believe he is "structurally" psychotic according to Kernberg's criteria. Also, he demonstrates several "forme fruste" examples of characteristic schizophrenic symptoms such as end-of-the-world fantasies and looseness of associations.

Unless otherwise noted, the remainder of the patient sample meets DSM-III-R criteria for schizophrenia (APA, 1987). When affective symptoms have been present, they have been brief in relation to the total duration of the disorder. In the pages that follow, I will provide a short synopsis of the histories of the patients who appear frequently in examples. Clearly, this is a heterogeneous group of patients, with a variety of strengths and disabilities. But that is consistent with the findings of years of research concerning diagnosis.

PATIENT SAMPLE

Mary Williams

Mary Williams was a 20-year-old woman from an impoverished city neighborhood. She was born to teenage parents who were poor and had little education. Her physical development was normal. Her psychiatric symptoms as a child included social isolation, self-injury, and aggressiveness. She was often afraid to be with other children, and often did not go to school, spending hours alone at neighborhood video arcades. As she got older, she became more verbally and physically aggressive and bizarre. Finally, in her midteens, she ran away from home, crossing the country from Illinois to Texas, where she lived in a shelter for runaways. At the time of her hospitalization in 1992, she was noted to have symptoms of depersonalization, derealization, looseness of association, tangentiality, circumstantiality, paranoid delusions (she thought her grandmother was a member of the Ku Klux Klan and intended to harm her) and auditory hallucinations (she heard the President talking to her). These symptoms had been present for two years, and had been treated without benefit with chlorpromazine 100 mg per day for several months before her hospitalization. The diagnosis made by several clinicians on admission was chronic undifferentiated schizophrenia according to DSM-III criteria. Psychological testing concluded that the patient had a "severe" loss of reality testing, a disturbed sense of boundaries, autistic and referential thinking, and that she felt that inanimate objects were alive.

It was not possible for the hospital staff to locate and contact the patient's family in Illinois and so no family history was available. A routine neurological exam revealed no abnormal findings. The patient was treated with fluphenazine 10 mg three times per day for the many months of her hospital stay. This was associated with a reduction of her auditory hallucinations, and delusions, but not of her thought disorder and bizarre behavior.

Ms. Williams was an inpatient and a day hospital patient at the time of the treatment described here. She had abused alcohol, marijuana, and phencyclidine in the past.

Deborah Weiss

Deborah Weiss was a 43-year-old Jewish woman from Colorado. She was raised by her parents and had one sister. There was no documented history of mental illness in her family. Her father was a high school teacher, and her mother worked as a receptionist. She attended a local community college, and after graduation, she took a job as a receptionist in an insurance firm. During this time, she had some friendships. Ms. Weiss had taken several trips to Israel and considered settling there, but ultimately, never did. She had been brought up as an Orthodox Jew, but became less observant as she got older. In her thirties, she was hospitalized for the first time, and never returned to work. Her functioning deteriorated progressively; over the course of the next thirteen years, she was hospitalized at least four times. Her symptoms included, at various times, auditory and visual hallucinations, persecutory and religious delusions, ideas of reference, depersonalization and derealization. Evidence of thought disorder included looseness of association, tangentiality, and pressured speech.

Most prominent when she was symptomatic were paranoid ideas concerning those closest to her and ideas of reference. She thought that she saw evidence of the imminent return of the

Messiah everywhere. When younger, she also had violent impulses which she struggled to control. She wanted to kill her boss and others who offended her. She stated that when she felt even a minor frustration, "my initial thought is to attack, but I hold myself back." Referring to her social isolation, she said, "There are cracks between people and me." Ms. Weiss complained bitterly of feeling dead, empty, and lethargic and thought that something must be wrong with her physically. An extensive neurologic workup which was undertaken was negative. This workup included a neurologic exam, a CAT scan of the head, a lumbar puncture, an electroencephalogram, blood work, and thyroid and viral studies.

Ms. Weiss did have episodes of aggressive excitement, but there was no clear history of manic symptoms. She often felt lethargic and without energy, but this was not connected to a well-defined depression. Her course was not episodic, and she never returned to her premorbid state. Treatment with lithium (1800 mg per day), tricyclic antidepressants (e.g., desipramine 250 per day for 2 months, and nortriptyline 100 mg per day for 2 months), MAO inhibitors (tranylcypromine sulfate 40 mg per day for 6 weeks), neuroleptics (e.g., haloperidol 10 mg per day for 4 months, and loxapine 150 mg per day for 3 months) and anxiolytics were minimally helpful.

Ms. Weiss had abused alcohol, stimulants, and morphine in the past, but was not taking these drugs at the time of the current treatment. She was diagnosed as having chronic paranoid schizophrenia by at least eight different clinicians using DSM-III and DSM-III-R criteria. No alternative diagnosis was proposed by any inpatient or outpatient facility. Ms. Weiss was an outpatient during the treatment described here.

Cathy Chen

Cathy Chen grew up in a suburban middle-class household in San Francisco. Her early development was relatively normal. There were six children in the home: three girls and three boys. Ms. Chen described her mother as a very competent woman. She was a member of the city council, and very active in city and state politics. Ms. Chen's father, an electrical engineer, was, by contrast, often withdrawn. There was some evidence of suspiciousness in the mother, and at times the father seemed disorganized, but no family member had ever been hospitalized, or taken psychiatric medication besides the patient.

Throughout her childhood and adolescence, the patient's mother imposed her unwelcome views upon her. Despite her love of sports, particularly swimming, her mother steered her toward a career in education. Despite paranoid thinking and social awkwardness, Ms. Chen was able to progress in school. After graduation, she went to work as a junior high school teacher.

Several years later, she had an acute decompensation. She came to believe that she was responsible for the serious illness of the governor of California. She believed that she and a prominent Chinese American newscaster were the same person. She had marked ideas of reference, and thought that her fellow teachers were sending surreptitious messages about her on the school public address system. She experienced the somatic delusion that she had a mastectomy. She believed literally that decomposing seaweed was all over her neck and back, and that termites were burrowing in her heart. She had frequent experiences of derealization and depersonalization, and complained of feeling lifeless and mechanical. She was very isolated socially. Her hospitalization occurred after an explosion of anger and incoherence during an airplane flight in which she intentionally hit her head on a door.

During her two-week hospitalization, she was noted to have looseness of association, ideas of reference, tangentiality, overabstract and concrete thinking, and inappropriate affect. She was treated successively with Triavil 4-25, two tablets three times per day for two months, and then haloperidol 20 mg per day for seven months following her hospital stay. The haloperidol treatment was associated with a reduction of auditory hallucinations and paranoid ideas. However, some paranoid ideas and ideas of reference, tangentiality, pressured speech, overabstract and concrete thinking, and inappropriate affect remained chronic despite neuroleptic treatment.

Ms. Chen did not have a history of depressive or manic symptoms, and her course was chronic. She was evaluated by a neurologist, and her neurologic exam and an electroencephalogram were within normal limits. Ms. Chen was diagnosed as having chronic paranoid schizophrenia according to DSM-III-R criteria by at least three clinicians. She did not abuse illegal drugs. She was an out-patient at the time of the psychotherapy described in this book.

Helen Jackson

Helen Jackson was a black woman in her early twenties who came from the rural South. The Jacksons had four children but, after a financial reversal, decided that they could no longer afford to raise them all. As an infant, the patient was sent to live with cousins, the Jordans. The patient lived with Mrs. Jordan until she was in high school, at which point Mrs. Jordan suffered a stroke and was institutionalized. Her biological parents were intermittently involved in the patient's life before Mrs. Jordan's institutionalization. As a child, the patient had some friendships, but as she got older, she became more socially isolated. Academically, she was able to do fairly well in high school, and took some computer training courses after graduation. She had a few short-lived relationships with men. Following this she worked at a series of unskilled jobs and her functioning deteriorated. This deterioration accelerated following the incapacitation of Mrs. Jordan. The patient began to act out. For example, while taking an aerobics class, she criticized the instructor for faulty technique and called the manager to have him removed. Following a financial disappointment, she became acutely psychotic. She was agitated, had grandiose delusions, and her behavior was disorganized. She showed evidence of looseness of association, tangentiality, circumstantiality, pressured speech, neologisms, and restricted, inappropriate, and blunted affect. She was admitted to the hospital on several occasions, where she stayed for a few months each time. She was treated with fluphenazine 20 mg per day for months with some improvement. Subsequently, as an outpatient, she was treated with loxapine succinate 800 mg per day for two months, and trifluoperazine 10 mg for three months, as well as a variety of other neuroleptics at unknown dosages. Antipsychotic treatment resulted in a decrease in agitation and bizarre behavior, but behavioral disorganization, looseness of association, pressured speech, and inappropriate affect remained chronic despite medication treatment.

The patient was evaluated as a young adult for headaches following an auto accident. Her neurological exam was normal as were skull X rays. A CAT scan revealed evidence of a "slight" concussion.

Ms. Jackson never had auditory hallucinations. She had no history of a depressive syndrome or manic symptoms. She denied a history of drug use. She was diagnosed in each hospital as having chronic undifferentiated schizophrenia according to DSM-III criteria. As an outpatient, she was also diagnosed as having schizophrenia. She was being treated as an outpatient during the period reviewed in this book.

Dorothy Hunt

Dorothy Hunt was a 25-year-old woman who came originally from the Midwest. She was raised by her grandfather, a retired widower, with the help of his unmarried sister, after her mother had abandoned her at 6 weeks of age. From childhood, Ms. Hunt was clearly different from other children, and acted in unpredictable and eccentric ways. She was teased and shunned by her peers. At the age of 20, she developed frank psychotic symptoms. She heard voices coming from the mailbox outside her home, which told her to kill her cousin, and she felt that her landlord had hired assassins to murder her. She thought that "music particles" had entered her clothes and believed that ghosts haunted her and that they exerted influence over her. She had prominent ideas of reference, inappropriate affect, and felt that thoughts became "ethereal substances" that were dangerous to her. On occasion, she rubbed her legs with sandpaper. On admission to the hospital, she was noted to have looseness of association, tangentiality, circumstantiality, thought blocking, and thought insertion.

The patient had no history of depressive or melancholic symptoms, or manic symptoms.

At least three different clinicians diagnosed chronic undifferentiated schizophrenia according to DSM-III-R criteria. Psychological testing noted an "absence of a feeling of reality" and concurred with the diagnosis of undifferentiated schizophrenia.

Despite numerous efforts, it was not possible to obtain a family history of psychiatric disorder from the patient's relatives. The patient had no history of drug abuse. No specific neurological evaluation was performed beyond a brief neurological exam, which was normal.

The patient was hospitalized on four occasions for several months at a time. She was treated with thiothixine 30 mg per day for four months, and trifluoperazine 30 mg per day for six weeks. These medications reduced agitation and auditory hallucinations, but did not eliminate the presence of pressured speech, tangentiality, circumstantiality, inappropriate affect, paranoid ideas or bizarre behavior.

Roger DeVito

Roger DeVito was an Italian man in his midthirties who had spent his childhood in Sicily. He came from a very large family of seven children, and, having five younger siblings, felt that his parents neglected him as a result. He recalled feeling empty inside since early childhood. Despite these troubles, he had a fairly good social adaptation and had a number of friendships as a child. The patient's parents died in a boating accident when he was 17, and he and several of his siblings lived with his aunt and uncle in the United States thereafter. He did well in school and eventually completed college and graduate school in accounting.

In his midtwenties, Mr. DeVito had the first of a series of numerous hospitalizations. His symptoms included prominent paranoid delusions. He believed that the head of a Mafia crime family somehow was living inside his heart, that his man controlled his behavior, and that he often spoke to the patient. He heard other voices which criticized him, and, on occasion, issued commands. "You will discover three of your family members murdered," they said, "and it will be because of you." Sometimes, Mr. DeVito would act bizarrely. On one occasion, he took a ferry to a remote island off the Oregon coast and wandered about until he was discovered by a park ranger. On another occasion, he built and erected a dozen religious statues in a downtown shopping mall. On several occasions, he was found in a catatonic posture, and would not speak.

Prominent among Mr. DeVito's chronic symptoms was a sense of inner deadness, alternating with emptiness. He felt that he was not the same as other people, that he lacked some essential human ingredient. He had some friends, but felt mechanical and dead with them.

Mr. DeVito's illness included some affective symptoms. At times, he became depressed, with poor sleep, poor appetite, and suicidal ideas. At other times, he seemed agitated and had increased energy and irritability. However, euphoria, increased talking, increased spending of money, racing thoughts, flight of ideas, the planning of new projects, and infectious likability were not prominent features of his illness.

Due to his affective symptoms, the diagnosis of bipolar affective disorder with psychotic features was made by several clinicians. However, it should be noted that Mr. DeVito's belief concerning the gangster who lived in his heart continued for years, and did not recede with the resolution of his affective symptoms. Moreover, there had been numerous episodes of psychotic symptomatology such as paranoid ideas, auditory hallucinations, and delusions, which occurred in the absence of any affective symptoms. The diagnosis in this case is not completely clear-cut, but it seems to me that the most accurate formulation is schizoaffective disorder according to DSM-III-R. Mr. DeVito was diagnosed variously as having schizophrenia, atypical psychosis, bipolar disorder with psychotic features, and schizoaffective disorder. In recent years, the most frequent diagnosis was schizoaffective disorder according to DSM-III-R. Psychological testing was done, and concluded, not surprisingly that the patient had a mixture of schizophrenic and affective symptoms.

Mr. DeVito had numerous psychiatric hospitalizations whose durations ranged from one to six months. He was treated with neuroleptics, inpatient electroconvulsive therapy (ECT), lithium carbonate, valproic acid, as well as antidepressants. Treatment with fluphenazine 30 mg per day for four months, lithium carbonate 2400 mg per day (with a blood level of 0.8 meq/L) for six months, and imipramine 200 mg per day for six weeks resulted in only modest benefit, and did not prevent the development of paranoid delusions, auditory hallucinations, or agitated behavior.

After several episodes of unresponsiveness the patient had an evaluation as an inpatient by a neurologist. He was noted to have a normal neurological exam with a normal CAT scan, MRI scan, and electroencephalogram.

The family reported schizophrenia in one first-degree relative. The patient did not use alcohol or illicit drugs.

Steven Tilden

Steven Tilden is a somewhat unusual member of this patient sample in that he was never hospitalized. Moreover, he never experienced acute psychotic symptoms such as auditory hallucinations, persistent delusions, or grossly disorganized behavior. Nevertheless, I think that including him in this study is justified.

Mr. Tilden was a 32-year-old man of Scottish heritage who lived in a large urban center in the Southeast. He was a tall, heavyset man with curly blond hair. He was raised in an urban middle-class home, and grew up in a very large family which included four sisters and four brothers. His mother was a chemistry professor and his father a physicist. He described his father as intensely involved with him in an often controlling way. His mother was intrusive, irritable, and sometimes frightening. Mr. Tilden's childhood was unremarkable except for a painful sense of isolation and disconnection from his peers.

The patient left home to attend college in Michigan where he continued to feel socially isolated. After graduation, he worked in various marketing jobs and lived on his own. He decided to begin psychotherapy after his girl friend of two months broke up with him.

When he started treatment, Mr. Tilden complained of intrusive preoccupations about his future success. Mostly, he thought about being an adored rock-and-roll star or being selected for promotion to a prominent position within his company. He also complained of problems in sorting out his thoughts, and that only a small portion of his mind was actually functioning. He felt that the phrases he chose to describe his thoughts and feelings were always "off the mark." His mind became "hollow" when he tried to accomplish an intellectual task. In addition, despite being an amateur bodybuilder who weighed over 220 pounds, he complained of feeling "lazy" and "unreal" in his legs and arms. He sometimes felt that people were going to attack him, but often was not certain that this was true.

Early in his psychotherapy, the patient was pleased that this therapist said little during the sessions. When the therapist spoke at a time the patient felt was inopportune, Mr. Tilden began a lengthy explanation that this behavior was not to be repeated. He believed that the therapist wanted to control him and make him "lifelessly" normal. When the therapist interpreted that the patient wished to control her, Mr. Tilden insisted even more that the therapist be quiet. On one occasion, when the therapist interpreted the patient's use of primitive projection, Mr. Tilden became agitated and walked out of the session.

In addition the patient often used idiosyncratic speech. He used private terms, some of which included Gaelic and Latin phrases and often seemed unaware that the therapist might not be able to translate this speech into conventional language. This translation could eventually be accomplished, but the patient's capacity to empathize with the therapist's position as a listener was limited.

At times of stress, Mr. Tilden seemed to have experiences similar to that of schizophrenic patients. When he began work after graduating college, he felt particularly lonely and shaky emotionally, and became preoccupied with the possibility of catastrophic earthquakes (unlikely events in Michigan). On another similar occasion, he became preoccupied with the thought that the destruction of the earth's ozone layer would accelerate leading to global destruction within a very short time. These concerns seemed to his therapist to be reminiscent of end-of-the-world fantasies described by schizophrenic patients. Mr. Tilden's sense of personal vulnerability was often intense.

The patient had occasional symptoms consistent with depression—some insomnia, crying, sadness, and lack of energy. However, these never met DSM-III-R criteria for Major Depression or Dysthymic Disorder.

Now, according to DSM-III-R, the patient might be diagnosed as having schizotypal personality disorder. Descriptively, this might be accurate. However, there is a question whether, according to Kernberg's criteria (1975, 1984), he can be diagnosed as having psychotic structure. As noted, when the therapist interpreted the patient's use of projective identification and omnipotent control, he became more suspicious, agitated, and disorganized. According to Kernberg, this suggests psychotic structure.

Since there are no external criteria to validate our current diagnostic schema objectively, the diagnosis of this man is a matter of debate. Despite this uncertainty, I include him in this work because even if not "overtly" schizophrenic, he appears to be a "form fruste" of psychosis, presenting embryonic forms of psychotic symptomatology, dynamics, and transference. As such, I believe his psychotherapy illustrates aspects of work with more frankly psychotic patients.

Mr. Tilden was treated at times with neuroleptics. He received trifluoperazine 5 mg per day, thiothixine 2 mg per day, and perphenazine 4 mg per day, each for several months, without apparent benefit. He had no formal neurological evaluation.

There was no history of major mental illness in the patient's first-degree relatives. The patient did not abuse alcohol or illegal drugs.

PSYCHOLOGY AND PSYCHOSIS

I would like to conclude this chapter on diagnosis by presenting two cases, which, I believe, illustrate important points about our assumptions concerning psychosis. Often we assume that psychotic symptoms must proceed from biological causes. We assume that such intense and wholesale disruptions of function are probably connected to physical disturbances in the "hard-wiring" of the nervous system and require equally physical forms of treatment such as medication and electroconvulsive therapy. When patients do not respond to treatment, and their psychotic symptoms get worse, we often take this as further evidence of the biological origin of the lesion. In other words, psychotic symptoms are "major" symptoms, and this means that they must have causes outside psychology and inside the body.

These assumptions may not be correct. We may encounter patients who demonstrate florid and bizarre forms of psychosis which do not respond to somatic treatments. When this occurs, we sometimes redouble our efforts to find a biological therapy only to find that the patient's condition persists or gets worse. In our effort to bring our most potent therapeutic weapons to bear, we often forget the power of psychology. Sometimes psychological work can accomplish what medication and ECT cannot.

In order to illustrate these points, I would like to present two brief case examples.

Michael Walker

Michael Walker was a 39-year-old Swedish-American man from the Midwest. He had a relatively normal childhood and adolescence with no evidence of psychiatric symptoms. He enjoyed good friendships and did well in school. He lived as an adult with his wife and five children. Mr. Walker had an episode of anxiety and depression in his early thirties which had been successfully treated with anxiolytics.

In his late thirties, the patient developed psychotic symptoms for the first time. These included auditory hallucinations, paranoid ideas, mutism and posturing, and were associated with such affective symptoms as sadness, lack of energy, anorexia, and insomnia. Mr. Walker reported that his father had been depressed for some time during his childhood, and that one of his brothers also suffered from depression. There was no history of drug or alcohol abuse. He was hospitalized and treated with thioridizine 100 mg per day for six weeks, and then trifluoperazine 50 mg per day for several months. His recovery was only partial and he was discharged feeling anxious and fragile.

Mr. Walker's decompensation had been associated with an intensifying estrangement from his wife. Mrs. Walker had been the victim of a sexual assault a year earlier, and had become severely inhibited sexually. Over the course of almost a year, the couple's sexual contact decreased markedly. Mr. Walker was interested in sexual relations, but his wife became progressively withdrawn until sexual relations stopped altogether.

About six months later, at the age of 39, Mr. Walker experienced an intensification of his symptoms. He began to see small figures, who he later identified as women, who stroked his hair and caressed his face. He saw apples and oranges on the floors of the house. These visual and tactile hallucinations were very disturbing to him. Despite treatment with lithium (1500 mg per day, with a blood level of 1.4 meq/L), thiothixene 40 mg per day, and sertraline hydrochloride 100 mg per day, these symptoms became so severe that the patient was rehospitalized. During the hospital stay, he had a neurological exam, an electroencephalogram, and a CAT scan, all of which were normal.

Mr. Walker remained in the hospital for many months. He was treated with loxitane 250 mg per day, and lithium carbonate 1500 mg per day (with blood levels of 1.5 meq/L). None of these treatments was dramatically effective, but over time, his symptoms diminished.

Following discharge from the hospital, the patient continued to have both somatic and visual hallucinations, and appeared fragile and confused. When he was alone, away from home, he would feel the presence of a tall woman, who would touch his face. He believed that this woman wanted sex, but her advances made him feel uncomfortable.

Two weeks after discharge, the patient began psychotherapy with Dr. W. The psychotherapy focused on Mr. Walker's intense longings for contact, and fear of isolation and loneliness. There were erotic feelings toward his female therapist as well which were also discussed. The patient's relationship with his wife was explored and he was able to acknowledge his feeling deprived of sexual contact with his wife. He expressed the fear that he would never really know sexual and romantic happiness.

In many respects, the work with Mr. Walker was slow and incomplete. Nevertheless, within five months, his symptoms abated almost completely. His visual, auditory, and tactile hallucinations which had at first persisted after discharge from the hospital now virtually ceased. Only the feeling that a woman caressed his face remained, and these episodes were very brief and intermittent. Mr. Walker was able to return to part-time employment. The patient's minute to minute preoccupation with his psychotic symptoms faded, and what symptoms remained he experienced as irritating rather than terrifying.

William Ishida

William Ishida was a man of Japanese ancestry. He grew up in a suburban town in Arizona. His mother worked outside the home and often left her children to the care of baby-sitters. The patient recalled feeling that he was not picked up or cuddled enough. The patient's father was a quiet and withdrawn man who did not play an active role in the care of the patient and his three younger sisters.

In his early thirties, the patient was treated for a number of depressive symptoms: sadness, anorexia, early morning awakening, diurnal mood variation, and suicidal thoughts. He was prescribed antidepressants and his symptoms gradually improved. During this time, he had episodes of trancelike states in which he seemed inaccessible, and other episodes in which he seemed overcome with emotion.

In his late thirties, Mr. Ishida married a somewhat older woman. Shortly after, she developed a chronic illness. The patient became her almost constant caretaker and sexual relations between the two were forsaken. Finally, his wife required hospitalization for an extended period of time. Within a few weeks, the patient became psychotic. He adopted rigid postures for long periods of time, became unresponsive, and heard voices telling him to harm himself in a variety of violent ways. He had experiences of derealization, and depersonalization and had visual hallucinations in which he saw worms crawling on his feet. During this time, Mr. Ishida had some depressive symptoms as well which included sadness, hopelessness, feeling slowed up, and the loss of emotion. He did not experience anorexia or diurnal mood variation. These symptoms continued on and off for several months. The patient was treated with nortriptyline 200 mg per day for six months, trifluoperazine 10 mg per day for six months, and lithium citrate 900 mg (with a blood level of 0.8 meq/L) for four months without much benefit. Finally, he was admitted to an acute care unit and was diagnosed as having a major depressive episode.

It was impossible to obtain a detailed family history of psychiatric illness. Mr. Ishida's family had returned to live in Japan many years before and were unavailable for interview. The patient maintained minimal contact with them and did not know the details of their medical histories. The patient denied alcohol or drug abuse. A neurological exam and an electroencephalogram several years before had both been normal.

After admission to the inpatient service, Mr. Ishida was given trifluoperazine 30 mg per day for over one month, followed by fluphenazine 20 mg per day for an additional six weeks. He also received desipramine 200 mg per day for a total of two months. None of these medications had an impact on the patient's symptoms. He was frequently placed in seclusion and had episodes of violent rage. He was preoccupied with aggressive and sexual images and fantasies and was terrified if anyone on the unit came too close. Finally after two months of medication treatment, the patient was transferred to a facility which emphasized psychotherapy as part of the treatment approach.

The patient's new psychiatrist, Dr. Keenan, began a twice per week psychotherapy which focused on the patient's affect. During the first few weeks, Mr. Ishida expressed enormous rage at the staff, the therapist, his wife, and his parents. Some of this was expressed rather incoherently, but some was comprehensible. The therapist interpreted that the patient's fear of closeness reflected a conflict: he had an intense longing for contact (i.e., to be held and caressed), but because of his fear of abandonment and his anger, he was afraid that contact would also lead to aggression and danger. Dr. Keenan interpreted that the patient was not sure whether he wanted to hug people or attack them.

Mr. Ishida began to relax his tense wariness within the first week of psychotherapy. Shortly, he was able to sit in a chair for a full session, and to express himself coherently. In addition to the themes of wished for contact and fear of violence, the next several weeks were spent exploring the patient's sexual concerns and frustrations.

Within several weeks of admission to the new facility, the patient was no longer psychotic. On a few occasions, for only minutes at a time, he experienced some hallucinations, but experiences quickly faded and the patient never again had psychotic symptoms. He continued his treatment in the hospital for several more weeks, and was then discharged. Mr. Ishida was able to remain nonpsychotic for at least a year and a half on follow-up.

Both Mr. Walker and Mr. Ishida were initially diagnosed by the inpatient staff as having an affective disorder, only to have this formulation revised when they did not respond to antidepressants, lithium, or electroconvulsive therapy. Subsequently, each was thought by different evaluators to be schizoaffective or schizophrenic.

One should note that it cannot be proven that the psychopathology in these two cases was resolved with psychological treatment. The temporal association of remission and psychotherapy is not conclusive. Nevertheless, these cases are significant for several reasons. First, it has been a rather widespread assumption that exploratory psychotherapy can undermine the fragile equilibrium of more disturbed patients. These cases suggest that even when patients have suffered from dramatic and long-standing psychosis, symptom reduction can be associated with psychological treatment. Even when extended and adequate trials of neuroleptics, lithium, and electroconvulsive therapy are not effective, psychological therapy may contribute to symptomatic improvement.

Second, these examples raise questions about whether "psychosis" is a product only of neuroanatomic or neurophysiologic factors. Psychological forces such as conflict connected to the need for affection, the need for sexual satisfaction, and the fear of one's own anger may be powerful enough in some individuals to stimulate a process which results in psychosis. From this standpoint, psychosis represents an endpoint to which not only the brain but the mind as well can lead. As I noted in the introduction, just as brain can move mind, so mind can move brain. If brain glucose metabolism can be changed following behavior therapy, and the anatomy and function of preoptic neurons in fish can be altered following social interaction, then it is reasonable to think that the image-forming apparatus can be modified by affect and cognition to result in such phenomena as hallucinations.

Finally, I would like to discuss a diagnostic issue. I have seen cases like the two presented above, in which psychological factors seemed to play a major role in the etiology of the disorder, and a significant role in its treatment. In some of these cases the duration of psychotic symptoms can be six months or longer. In a number of these patients there is a history of early childhood trauma, often sexual abuse. Premorbid functioning is often good. Patients have done well in school and work, and are able to establish significant friendships. When the psychosis appears, symptoms can include delusions, ideas of reference, paranoid ideas, auditory, visual, and tactile hallucinations, bizarre behavior and ideas, mutism, posturing, and disturbances of affect.

Often, floridly psychotic patients do not seem to be schizo-phrenic. As noted, premorbid social and vocational adjustment is often good. They do not show the extreme brittle fragility in their object relations that is characteristic of schizophrenic pa-tients who can end years' long relationships in a snap. There is no long-term impoverishment of affect or thought, although in the short term there can be what appears to be flattening of affect or loosening of associations. The disturbance in their symbolic functioning is transitory, and the link between dynamic conflict and the impairment of symbol use is more apparent and clear-cut. Moreover, this group of patients differs from schizophrenics in that they appear to respond relatively rapidly to psychological intervention. Interpretation, even inexact interpretation of rela-tively superficial layers of conflict, can often be associated with rapid and marked improvement; this is not the case with patients who are schizophrenic.

In view of the importance of this diagnostic category and the importance of distinguishing it from schizophrenia, I would suggest that it be given a separate name. It is relatively immaterial what name is used. One might use the term *psychogenic psychosis* to emphasize the importance of psychological factors in the etiol-ogy and treatment of the disorder. Equally well, one might use the term *hysterical psychosis.* This term links the disorder to similar groups of patients that other investigators (Hollender and Hirsch, 1964; Hirsch and Hollender, 1969; Siomopoulus, 1971; Spiegel and Fink, 1979) have described, and emphasizes the presence of such "hysterical" phenomena as fugue states, sexual fantasies and trauma, disturbances of perception, flamboyant somatic symp-tomatology, and displays of affect. It also establishes a link to the patients whom Freud treated early on, who had florid visual and somatic symptoms associated with psychodynamic conflict.

My purpose is not to claim that a large portion of patients whom we classify as schizophrenic in fact suffer from "hysterical psychosis," and should therefore be treated only with psychother-apy in the expectation of a rapid and dramatic cure; that is not at all the case. I simply seek to emphasize the importance of paying careful attention to psychological factors whenever psycho-sis occurs. If we do not give psychological forces adequate atten-tion, not only may we miss an opportunity to use psychological interventions for the benefit of truly schizophrenic patients, but we may overlook the diagnosis and treatment of a category of patients which responds especially well to psychotherapy. There have been cases in which the patient's lack of response to somatic therapy signaled to the staff that they faced a truly tenacious biological illness, and the effort at somatic treatment was redoubled only to exacerbate the patient's condition. Unfortunately psychotherapy often is considered either irrelevant or actually pernicious in these cases of "major psychosis." Even though this group may include a relatively small percentage of patients with long-standing and dramatic psychotic symptoms, it would be unfortunate to overlook an effective treatment.

Chapter 2

Comparison with Other Techniques

$\mathbf{I}$would briefly like to compare the psychotherapy techniques I am describing in this book to some of the best known approaches to the psychotherapy of schizophrenia. I think that this will help me to be more precise in my description of various techniques, and why I think they are particularly suited to work with patients who have a psychotic structure.

Mainstream psychoanalysis followed Freud's lead in avoiding the use of psychoanalytic techniques with schizophrenic patients. Among Freud's objections to psychoanalytic work with schizophrenics, was his belief that schizophrenic patients were not able to establish the transference upon which psychoanalytic work depended. He wrote (1916–1917), "Observation shows that sufferers from narcissistic neuroses have no capacity for transference or only insufficient residues of it. They reject the doctor, not with hostility but with indifference. For that reason they cannot be influenced by him either; what he says leaves them cold, makes no impression on them; consequently the mechanism of cure which we carry through with other people cannot be operated with them" (p. 447).

Paul Federn was a notable exception to the general psychoanalytic pessimism concerning work with schizophrenic patients (1934, 1943a,b,c, 1952). He used psychoanalytic techniques in his work with schizophrenic patients, albeit in a modified and limited way. Federn emphasized the importance of helping the patient maintain a positive transference. His goal was to encapsulate the psychosis and to strengthen the nonpsychotic part of the patient's personality. To accomplish this, he advocated the abandonment of free association, analysis of the positive transference, and of

41

the analysis of resistance and defense. He also advocated suspending the treatment if the negative transference grew too intense.

More recently Arlow and Brenner (1964, 1969) have argued that neurosis and psychosis exist on a continuum, and that the symptoms of psychosis no less that those of neurosis arise as a result of conflict, defense, and compromise formation. They present a theory of psychotic psychopathology in which symptoms serve as defenses against intense anxiety and guilt. In their view, one of the unique features of psychosis is that there is a regression in the functioning of the ego in the service of defense. In particular, defensive modifications of the ego's capacity to integrate mental contents, and to use language, impair the functioning of the schizophrenic patient. They advocate the use of interpretation to ameliorate the effects of this ego regression.

Boyer and Giovachini (1967, 1980) claim to have treated schizophrenic patients with the use of unmodified psychoanalysis. They recommend the use of the couch and free association. They believe that the treatment falls into two phases. In the first, or "noisy phase" the goal is to replace cold, hostile internal objects with warm, loving ones. This is done by making contact with the patient through verbal interpretation, and by maintaining a hopeful, optimistic, detached attitude. In the noisy phase the patient's distortions, contradictions, and abandonments of reality are gently confronted. The defensive function of their use of psychotic thinking is interpreted and there is a focus on aggressive drive derivatives. A second phase of treatment follows in which a transference neurosis is established and interpreted.

Boyer and Giovachini believe that there is a striving in the psychotic patient toward ego maturation, and that the working through of the regressive psychotic transference reduces conflict and enables the maturation of conflict-free aspects of ego functioning. They emphasize the centrality of interpretation as a method both for making contact with the patient and effecting a revision of faulty ego and superego structures.

One problem with the work of Boyer and Giovachini is the nature of their patient sample. They exclude patients who are "chronically regressed" and warn against the treatment of patients with paranoid schizophrenia. Many of their patients are described as depressed with psychoses following childbirth, manic, hypomanic, borderline, and schizoaffective. It is not at all clear how ill the patients in their sample are; whether they suffer from schizophrenia, affective disorders (with the accompanying spontaneous remissions to intact functioning), or severe character disorders.

Moreover, Boyer and Giovachini define psychosis after Bychowski (1957, p. 129) as being characterized by magical and concrete thinking, primitive introjection and projection, and primary identification, and the use of splitting mechanisms. This constitutes a "psychotic core" and is characterized by dyadic transferences. When triadic transferences emerge, the authors consider this to be evidence that the core of the patient's psychopathology is no longer psychotic. They also use the results of psychological testing to assess the degree of change in their patients.

Boyer and Giovachini do not describe treatment with regressed patients. It is not at all clear that the patients they describe are schizophrenic or that those who in fact were psychotic (and did not have character disorders) did not suffer primarily from affective disorders which may improve over the course of time without treatment. Moreover, the presence of triadic elements in the transference is not, I believe, unique to patients who are neurotic, and does not in itself establish the resolution of psychotic structure.

Another important approach to the psychotherapy of schizophrenic patients was begun by Sullivan (1940, 1953, 1962, 1964). He believed that schizophrenic patients do, in fact, establish transferences, even if they are often intense and unstable. He described what he called the "one genus hypothesis" (1953, pp. 32–33) which emphasized that schizophrenic patients are more like other human beings than they are different. He emphasized that the symptoms of schizophrenia resulted from the patient's flight from anxiety and his need for security. Sullivan emphasized the importance of establishing contact with schizophrenic patients, and the need to approach the often frightened and traumatized patient with respect, tolerance, and acceptance. In an effort to make such contact, departures from traditional analytic neutrality and detachment were often necessary. The therapist functioned as a "participant observer." The therapist might, for example, communicate his own feelings to the patient if that helped to make a human connection. It was essential to be honest in one's interactions with the patient.

Frieda Fromm-Reichmann (1959) followed Sullivan's lead in emphasizing the importance of the patient–therapist relationship. She emphasized the patient's defensive escape from pain, conflict, and anxiety. At first, she believed that the schizophrenic patient suffered from powerful narcissistic injuries and that it was essential that the therapist help foster a positive relationship with the patient. Later, she came to feel that one must not ignore the patient's aggression and must address it in the psychotherapy. She felt that if the therapist tries to discourage the expression of aggression, the patient believes this to be evidence of the therapist's fear of his own or the patient's hostility.

Working within this tradition, Elvin Semrad (Semrad, Menaer, Mann, and Standish, 1952; Semrad, 1966) believed that psychotic symptoms represented maladaptive behavior. He saw therapy as a "corrective ego experience" in which the therapist might have to be "gratifying, rewarding and growth stimulating" in order to help the schizophrenic patient. He wrote that therapeutic interventions might involve "gratifying needs, and providing sustenance, support and security, as long as the study of the patient's flights is in process" (1966, p. 159). Semrad believed that the basis of the patient's symptoms was a flight from unpleasure which overwhelmed the ego, and led to a "body response to disintegration, terror, fear, panic and dread." He emphasized that the treatment was an intimate experience in which the therapist needed to feel many of the painful affects from which the patient was trying to escape. The essential work of the treatment was to help the patient to "acknowledge, bear and keep in perspective" (p. 157) painful affects and painful life experiences, often connected to loss. The therapist needed to help the patient "stop, look, listen, and stop running." The patient's developing ability to tolerate such affects and to put them into words was the bedrock of his improvement.

Another important approach to the psychotherapy of schizophrenia was begun by Melanie Klein (1923, 1930, 1935, 1946, 1957). Klein described two principal emotional "positions" in early childhood to which adult psychotic patients regressed: the schizoid position and the depressive position. The schizoid position was characterized by paranoid anxieties about physical and emotional attack, cycles of projected and introjected aggression, fantasies of the self splitting into fragments and entering others and being subsequently reintrojected, and object relations characterized by part objects. Part objects were understood to be representations of the self and others in which parts of the physical or emotional self are split off or isolated from other parts of the self. An image of an exclusively "good" mother who is somehow uncontaminated by fantasies about the "bad" aspects of the mother is an example. In the depressive position, the affects of hate and love are integrated and result in the capacity for guilt and concern. Guilt springs from anxiety about the harm that one's aggression can bring to those whom one loves. The capacity to integrate love and aggression ushers in the possibility of whole object relations in which self and object representations are characterized by both "good" and "bad" aspects.

The relations between the schizoid position and the depressive are complex. The achievement of the depressive position signals not only a maturational step, but also a method of resolving paranoid anxieties by establishing more loving and constant object relations which can withstand the onslaught of aggression. At the same time, if depressive anxieties become overwhelming, there may be a defensive regression to the schizoid position as a defense against guilt.

Hanna Segal (1950, 1964) was one of the first within the Kleinian tradition to write specifically about psychotherapy with schizophrenic patients. She emphasized the role of splitting and denial as well as introjective and projective mechanisms in psychopathology. She said that unlike in neurosis in, psychosis, a great deal of primitive fantasy was conscious, but that the links between fantasies, and the links between fantasy and reality were repressed.

Segal applied Kleinian principles of interpretation to schizophrenic patients and felt that it was important to "interpret the unconscious material at the level of the greatest anxiety, much as I would do with a neurotic" (1950, p. 113). In practice, for Kleinian analysts working with schizophrenic patients this often means identifying an intense anxiety, related to primitive body-related fantasies. Klienian analysts believe that these fantasies often involve projection and introjection of such bodily contents as feces, urine, and semen, or such mental contents as ideas and emotions.

These contents are often felt to be evacuated into the other, controlling them from the inside. Parts of the physical, emotional, or mental self are thereby lost, and the schizophrenic feels emptied and barren. There may also be fantasies of attack by the other, in which these often "bad" parts of the self are violently forced back. Primitive anxieties include the fear of falling into bits, or being driven crazy by the attempts of the other to force his bad aspects into the patient. The role of the analyst is to make these primitive and rather complex fantasies conscious by interpretation. Segal gives an example of an interpretation made to a schizophrenic man who had auditory hallucinations and had started to practice eye exercises.

> Then I made a more complete interpretation. I reminded him of the death of his two relatives, his identification with them, his refusal to mourn them, and the triumph over them during the weekend. I suggested that, in performing eye exercises, he was watching the intercourse between his parents, and that he was killing the father or both parents, presented by the two relatives, by magic looking and magic counting. Finally he introjected the dead and triumphed over them. But apparently, they were not defeated; they came back to life inside him and mocked him, mocked particularly his magic looking and counting—the means by which, he thought, he had secured his triumph [1950, pp. 107–108].

It is difficult for the reader to make a judgment about how well this formulation is supported by the previous associative material, because Segal does not go into detail.

Segal also emphasized the disruption of symbolic thinking in schizophrenic patients and its role in such symptoms as concrete thinking and disturbed language use.

Rosenfeld (1952, 1954, 1965, 1969, 1987) also used Kleinian concepts in his work with schizophrenic patients. He emphasized the importance of paying "minute attention to the patient's communications" (1987, p. 4). Like Segal, he advocated interpreting the patient's "most prominent immediate anxiety" (p. 40). Rosenfeld emphasized the central importance of the countertransference as a guide to the patient's inner state. Using projective identification, rather than verbal symbols, the schizophrenic patient conveys information to the therapist about his inner states. At times, feelings stirred up in the therapist may provide the only clues as to what is going on in the patient.

Like Segal, Rosenfeld described complex interpretations which identified intense anxieties and primitive fantasies. He wrote of a Dr. O, working from a Kleinian perspective. Sarah, the patient, had apparently wished to deny her need to depend on the analyst. She said, "But you are a fool for peddling dope, you could be outside doing it with oxygen." Rosenfeld reports:

> Dr. O. had established that this oxygen had for some time been a symbol for semen. He felt the material, therefore, indicated there was suddenly a confusion in Sarah's mind about the relationship of the breast, nipple and penis. In the session before, there had been references to oxygen and to the sexual relationship between the parents, so he tried to differentiate between the confusion in the baby's mind. Her baby self is centred between the nipple, which comes into her mouth and on which she feels dependent but which she confuses with her addiction to masturbation, and her father's penis, which is felt at the weekend to be going into the mother's mouth to feed and restore her. Her demand, "You could be doing it outside with oxygen," therefore, refers to her baby self claiming that the penis could serve her in a much better way, without the dependence on the analytic nipple [1987, p. 233].

According to Rosenfeld, this is Dr. O's formulation and presumably also his verbal intervention with the patient.

Like Segal, Rosenfeld also emphasizes the loss of symbol use in schizophrenia. He connects disturbed symbol use to "excessive projective identification (with its massive creation of objects fused with the self) [which] interferes with symbolization and verbal thinking . . ." (1987, p. 229). Rosenfeld stresses the importance of interpreting projective identification and splitting within the treatment in order to preserve verbal thinking. However, as intriguing as these links are between the loss of symbol use and these primitive defenses, Rosenfeld only alludes to the mechanism by which they may be connected. He does not give an explicit account.

Rosenfeld's very interesting account of his work with schizophrenic patients shares a problem mentioned earlier. He does not provide enough information about the patient sample for the reader to determine for himself whether these patients are in fact schizophrenic. The patient "Sylvia" is described as having a "breakdown" and as "mentally collapsed" (1987, p. 45). Iris is a "young unmarried woman of twenty five [who] was in the throes of her third schizophrenic attack" (1987, p. 222). Sarah "had been manifestly schizophrenic for five months, prior to which she had been in acute psychotic depression for two-and-a-half years, having been hospitalized and given ECT on two occasions" (1987, p. 224).

Thomas Ogden (1982) has also written from the perspective of Kleinian theory. He emphasized the central role of projective identification as a primitive form of communication by the patient. The therapist must be open to the affects and fantasies stirred up by the patient as offering clues to his inner life. Ogden described various stages in the therapeutic work with schizophrenic patients in which the patient first makes use of projective identification, and only later verbal symbols to communicate about his thoughts and feelings. Like Rosenfeld, Ogden did not provide detail about his patients' symptom histories, and so it is hard to judge which patients were in fact schizophrenic.

I would like to make a few brief comments about how the techniques presented in this book resemble and differ from those of the three broad traditions presented above.

My own approach is similar to that of the psychoanalytic theorists in that it emphasizes the defensive nature of many schizophrenic phenomena. It relies on clarification, confrontation, and interpretation of the patient's material. I believe that the interpretation of conflict can ameliorate at least some aspects of schizophrenic psychopathology.

My approach differs in that I do not believe that neurosis and schizophrenia occupy a continuum, differentiated only by degree or intensity. I think that the psychological structure of schizophrenia differs fundamentally from that of neurosis. The functions of the ego, in particular, symbol use, in schizophrenia

are profoundly different from that in neurosis. Because psychotherapy is such an exquisitely verbal event, one must first address
distortions of symbol use before one can undertake a standard
verbal treatment. Authors within the traditional psychoanalytic
tradition do not seem to address this problem.

My approach draws a great deal from that of Sullivan and
his followers. Their emphasis on the importance of the therapist–patient relationship, especially the importance of treating
the patient as a respected colleague in the therapeutic work, is
very valuable. I agree with Semrad (1966) and Searles (1962,
1963, 1965, 1971, 1972) that one must often experience very
primitive and painful affects, such as emptiness, hopelessness, and
meaninglessness if one is to remain in contact with a schizophrenic patient. Work with such patients requires a great deal of
emotional effort. I also agree that in the service of acknowledging
the accuracy of the patient's reality testing, it is important to be
candid and honest with the patient about one's thoughts and
feelings. Not to reveal aspects of oneself at certain moments may
confirm the patient's fear that such feelings are too painful to
bear and frightening to talk about.

Like writers in the Sullivanian tradition, I think it is crucial
to work with the patient to identify and verbalize their inner
states. In work with a regressed schizophrenic patient one must
often start with helping him attach words to sensations, affects,
fantasies, and ideas. No further psychotherapy is possible if the
patient does not have a lexicon for his inner states. Semrad's
emphasis on the need to help the patient become aware of his
inner life, despite the considerable pain this generates, is essential.

Writers from the Interpersonal School, however, are often
not specific about technique. Like the traditional psychoanalytic
theorists, schizophrenic psychopathology is understood to exist
on a continuum with neurosis. Specific differences in ego functioning and language use are not emphasized.

Kleinian analysts have contributed an enormous amount to
work with schizophrenic patients. Their descriptions of primitive
defenses such as splitting, projective identification, and denial
have been very helpful. Their emphasis on the differences between paranoid–schizoid anxieties and depressive concerns has
also been very important. Their account of the role of primitive

object relations and affects such as envy, contempt, devaluation, and idealization have helped clarify a number of important transference phenomena. And the emphasis upon the use of countertransference as a guide to the internal life of the schizophrenic patient (Racker, 1968) who verbally is out of contact is crucial.

However, my approach differs from these Kleinian authors in several ways. Unlike theorists from the perspective of traditional ego psychology, the Kleinian analysts discussed (with the exception of Ogden) do not appear to interpret from "surface to depth." They do not direct their interpretations at the surface of the material, focusing either on affect or resistance, and work so that deeper material unfolds gradually. Rather, they direct their interpretations to what seems to be the deepest or most intense or most primitive anxieties associated with the patient's fantasy. Their interventions seem to focus on introjective and projective mechanisms connected with primitive fantasies about body parts and contents. These interventions seem to have a somewhat stereotyped and arbitrary quality, and do not seem to spring from the patient's particular associations. I am concerned not only that these interpretations may not be accurate, but that they do not sufficiently account for the patient's need for a "psychic surface," that is, a cognitive realm which is *not* so immediately connected to what is primitive in the patient. If concept and symbol formation is to occur, it must take place in a "mental realm" which has boundaries and integrity of its own, and exists separately from body organs and physiological states. To deemphasize surface material in schizophrenic patients and focus so consistently on what is "deep" or "primitive" may be to undermine the patient's need to erect a repressive barrier between conscious and unconscious, between secondary process and primary process. To make this point is *not* to embrace Federn's suggestion that we ignore or encapsulate what is psychotic in the patient. Rather, it is to acknowledge that the schizophrenic patient needs an intact surface as well as a vital depth, and that one must proceed gradually from one to the other.

Related to this point is the use of complex verbal interventions by a number of Kleinian analysts. In the examples I have given, the analyst makes lengthy and complicated statements to the patient. To understand and make use of these interventions requires considerable cognitive skills including attention, concentration, memory, and a facility for class concept use. We know that schizophrenic patients have profound troubles especially in these areas. To make such interpretations, we must assume that there exists a nonpsychotic part of the personality which remains intact, kind of verbally sophisticated homunculus, in which these verbal skills remain preserved, and which can attend to and integrate complex interpretations. I think that this is a very questionable notion. What this nonpsychotic part of the personality is actually like in any particular patient is very unclear. It may be adept at symbol use, or it may not. It may suffer from some of the same difficulties in symbol use as its psychotic counterpart. It may play a large role in overall ego functioning, or only a small one. Even if we are optimistic, and assume that alongside the psychotic ego, there exists an ego which is completely normal, and in which all the essential ego functions are preserved, that does not mean that such an ego could assimilate the lengthy and complex interpretations offered by some Kleinian analysts. There are many verbally sophisticated neurotic patients in psychoanalysis, who cannot assimilate verbally complicated interventions.

Finally, I think that some Kleinian analysts who work with schizophrenic patients approach the therapeutic task as if the analyst were a kind of codebreaker, and the patient a codemaker. The patient presents verbally obscure and complex material and it is the therapist's job to decode it. While some of these decodings may be accurate, they call upon the therapist to make virtuoso performances of translation. Moreover, they do not address the way in which patient and therapist have become engaged in the codemaking–codebreaking process. My own view is that it would be better for the therapist to remain "naive" in his stance, to not assume too much of an understanding based on translations of obscure symbols, but to point out to the patient that he is being obscure. To not do this, in many cases, is to undermine the patient's reality testing. If an average social observer cannot understand what the patient is saying then he needs to know this. If the patient needs a trained analyst familiar with primitive fantasies to understand him, then there is certainly something amiss in the way he communicates. It is important to point out these problems in communication not only to help the patient appreciate the social reality of the interaction, but to begin an exploration of the defensive functions that his obscurity may have. My approach attempts to address this issue.

Chapter 3

Structuring the Treatment

While the ultimate goal of psychotherapy with schizophrenics is to reduce symptoms and their devastating effects, clearly this cannot be achieved quickly. Medication and organic forms of treatment usually take time to produce results, and this is all the more true for psychotherapy. Also, psychotherapy is not something that can begin at once. It is a process which both parties must learn to do together.

Work with patients who have severe character disorders has shown that patients may not be able at the outset to participate in verbal psychotherapy. In fact, they may not know what psychotherapy really consists of. Borderline patients often translate feeling into action rather than words. Self-destructive impulses may find their way into self-cutting, neglect of essential medical treatments, inattention to work or school deadlines, and so on. Moreover, even verbalizations in psychotherapy can constitute "acting out." Kernberg (1975) cites the example of a patient who yelled at her therapist during session after session. He concluded that this was not "working through," but rather a repetitive gratification of aggressive wishes. When the therapist told the patient to stop, for the first time anxiety and concern appeared.

Borderline patients require modified psychoanalytic technique, in part because, unlike neurotics, they cannot follow the "fundamental rule" of psychoanalysis. Because they rely so much on splitting as a defense, confrontation is far more necessary than with neurotics. The consequences of splitting involve a more necessary part of the work bringing to consciousness areas of awareness that have been kept apart. And because these patients express so much in action, setting up parameters (Eissler, 1953a;

53

Kernberg, 1975) and setting limits are also more central to the treatment. These steps are taken in order to preserve the *verbal* nature of the treatment. A treatment that does not call upon the patient to verbalize rather than to act is not psychotherapy. If impulses are gratified rather than spoken, understanding cannot occur. Limits on the patient's behavior, then, may be set in order: (1) to preserve his safety (a hospitalized or severly injured patient cannot participate in psychotherapy); (2) to preserve a minimum level of calm and equanimity so that the therapist can think and feel freely; and (3) to channel powerful affect and hard-to-tolerate thought into comprehensible words, rather than incomprehensible action.

These challenges to establishing a verbal psychotherapy in borderline patients are even greater in work with schizophrenics, whose speech is often incomprehensible, and who use words as often as not to obscure as to help in communicating. Not only is the verbal apparatus dismantled in many of these patients (it is not clear whether this is a result of biological or psychological processes), but so also is their capacity to think in concepts. They not only want to conceal conscious feelings from others, and to abolish painful feelings from their own awareness, but often the mechanism for conceptualizing feelings in itself is impaired. In other words, the capacity of these patients to symbolize is frequently lost. They do not have a language for their inner states. They may transform concepts and ideas into sensations, and thus remove themselves from the conceptual or verbal realm.

As if this were not enough, these patients have a devastating impairment in their capacity to maintain a relationship. Deeply vulnerable to the loss of self-esteem, and longing profoundly for closeness to the point of fantasied merger and fusion, and deathly afraid of their own rage and the retaliation of others, they can break off treatment for good with little notice. The fear of their own aggression is compounded by their inability to distinguish between themselves and others. Thus, rageful fantasies of attack are not contained within themselves, permitting the therapist to remain a helping ally. The clinician then is perceived to be dangerous, and the patient contemplates fight or flight. Such fantasies inevitably poison the image of the therapist. Accepting an "interpretation" from such a dangerous therapist requires a faith and freedom from suspiciousness that these patients do not yet have.

Sometimes such patients may try to control the therapist's behavior and speech to protect themselves from frightening amounts of their own envy, rage, and anxiety. This may leave the therapist with the unfortunate options of remaining silent, leaving essential material undiscussed, or speaking up and precipitating flight.

Schizophrenic patients will often deny the realistic consequences of their actions in the outside world, and disrupt treatment by getting themselves hospitalized, arrested, or cut off financially from supportive family. They may spend such vast amounts of time in unrealistic activities or isolated fantasy states, that no psychotherapy relationship can compete for access to their inner worlds. Such "autistic" states may be deeply gratifying. They permit the fantasy that the patient has escaped his "mortal coil" and is not subject to the same limits of time, space, death, and loss as his fellows. From such a perch, what would induce a patient to reenter the mundane world and discover the true outlines of his social, cognitive, and emotional impairment? To say that such a patient "lacks motivation" for psychotherapy is a profound understatement.

Schizophrenic patients can disrupt their psychotherapies by making themselves so offensive and obnoxious to the therapist, that he can only think of ridding himself of his burden. The patient can make the therapist feel impotent, empty, dead, fraudulent, immoral, self-centered, frightened, crazy, enraged, or revolted. In the best of circumstances, such countertransference affects are conscious and the therapist has a fighting chance to deal with them. Often, however, many operate unconsciously, and may lead the therapist to find a rationale to have the patient treated elsewhere.

In order for any psychotherapy to work, several essentials must be in place: (1) The patient must be able to come; (2) he must have a wish to tell his story to someone who will listen; (3) he must have the conceptual wherewithal to do so, that is, he must be able to put his ideas and feelings into words; (4) he must have financial resources, or the support of those who do; (5) he must find someone willing to make sense out of what he says; and (6) he must refrain from attacking the physical setting or the composure of the listener so that the latter can pay attention to what the patient has to say.

The task of the therapist is to create conditions necessary for a verbal psychotherapy. He does this by identifying the factors that prevent this from happening. Some of these, such as the patient's disturbances in symbolization and in the self-object boundary, can be ameliorated only slowly, over time. Some, such as the patient's yelling, refusing to take medication, sleeping twenty hours a day, can and should be addressed at the outset. The purpose of this chapter is to outline some principles which can be used to structure verbal psychotherapy with schizophrenic patients.

There are generally three ways in which the patient can disrupt the basic conditions for psychotherapy:

1. The patient's behavior so gratifies (usually split-off) impulses that he is unwilling to examine them psychologically (Kernberg, 1975). This may occur if the patient verbally abuses the therapist, threatens harm, damages physical property, uses drugs, and so on.
2. The patient's behavior so alienates, disturbs, frightens, stimulates, or disrupts the therapist that he or she is either unable or unwilling to maintain technical neutrality, or even to listen to the patient at all.
3. The patient's behavior destroys his ability to attend sessions. This may be accomplished by alienating supporting family members, destroying sources of income or insurance coverage, or by spending long stretches of time in the hospital.

What follows will focus mainly on outpatient treatment. Some of what I will say follows Kernberg's (1975, 1984) suggestions concerning the psychotherapy of borderlines.

I would like to begin with a case example which illustrates many of the problems of outpatient treatment with schizophrenic patients. Helen Jackson came for treatment at the request of her grandparents. Ms. Jackson was orphaned when her mother, who had been divorced from her father, died during the patient's infancy. Following this, after a brief spell in foster care she had been sent to live with cousins, the Jordans, as an infant. She lived with the Jordans until Mrs. Jordan had a stroke and was institutionalized when the patient was in her midtwenties. Following this, she lived for a time with her aunt and uncle, the Tafts, in a rural community. The patient had been hospitalized on many occasions for auditory hallucinations, paranoid and grandiose ideas, bizarre behavior, and poor self-care. She had graduated from high school, but had trouble keeping simple jobs. Nevertheless, she believed that, one day, she would become a well-known and successful businesswoman. She had a profound thought disorder, with marked loosening of associations, and marked tangentiality. Her affect was very often inappropriate and restricted. She was not easy to live with. Her behavior was frequently very primitive. While living with the Tafts, she would throw garbage out of the window on the lawn and throw her dirty laundry out on the street.

The Tafts anticipated problems with the arrival of the patient. On the advice of their pastor, they arranged for Ms. Jackson to see a therapist soon after she settled in. Although it was unstated, part of their motive was to prevent their niece from being a "behavior problem." Because of powerful feelings of family obligation, they felt unable to refuse her request to live with them, but clearly feared that her presence would upset their usual way of living. At the beginning, Ms. Jackson's uncle was willing to provide transportation for her to attend twice per week psychotherapy. This represented a considerable commitment since it took about twenty minutes each way by car, and public bus or train service did not exist between the patient's home and the therapist's office.

For her part, the patient was unsure whether she wanted to live with the Tafts whom she thought had little time for her, or to return to live with vaguely identified friends. She got the message that her aunt and uncle wanted her to be in better control. She attended her psychotherapy sessions, but soon expressed a wish that she and the therapist make her quickly "recovered" so that she could leave town and return to live with her friends. She wanted to get on with her plans to get a job and succeed in the business world.

The patient began her tenth session by walking into a group run by a colleague of the therapist's in another office in the suite. Ms. Jackson grudgingly left after the group leader asked her to do so. Her therapist, Dr. S, later explained that the work with the group was private, and that she could not enter offices other than her therapist's. The therapists in the suite needed to safeguard the privacy of all the patients as well as that of Ms. Jackson, she explained.

Several times during this period, the patient removed journals and books stored in a closet next to the waiting room. Dr. S advised her to return the material and asked about why she had taken it. Ms. Jackson answered that she was curious, and laughed. The therapist then told her that this made her angry, and that Ms. Jackson was treating her things as if they were her own. If they were going to meet, Dr. S said, then the patient would have to stop this. The therapist also wanted to discuss why Ms. Jackson had acted as she had. They discussed Ms. Jackson's feeling that she was a burden to her relatives, and her envy of the therapist.

As time went on, the patient and therapist were able to do much productive work. Progressively, the patient was able to put her feelings of failure, isolation, loneliness, emptiness, rage, and envy into words. Despite various disappointments and outbursts of rage at Dr. S, the patient persevered.

The therapist had explained to the patient and her family that it was essential that Ms. Jackson have some structured therapeutic activity during the day, such as a training program or day hospital, so that the psychotherapy not bear the entire brunt of the patient's treatment needs. She also explained that psychotherapy was not the answer to all of Ms. Jackson's problems. The patient and her family agreed. For weeks afterwards, Ms. Jackson told her therapist that she was attending an agricultural work program which was training her for a farm job, and which in fact, she had applied to.

Within a short time, the structure of the psychotherapy began to crumble. The Tafts reported that after several weeks of good participation in the farm training program, the patient had stopped attending. When confronted with this, the patient dismissed the significance of both her failure to attend and her lying about it. Also, Mr. Taft, who was responsible for driving the patient to the session, began to complain of the inconvenience. This seemed to represent some unspoken criticism of the psychotherapeutic treatment. The patient began to talk increasingly about the need for speedy treatment, and her wish to return to live in the South. When she was asked, she acknowledged that her uncle said it was hard for him to do so much driving.

Suddenly, Mr. Taft told the patient to stop her sessions, and the patient called Dr. S to end the treatment.

The above account is a very incomplete summary of all that went on, and leaves out much of the details of the psychotherapeutic work. More of the work in this case will be presented in later chapters. Nevertheless, this vignette illustrates a number of problems one encounters in setting up psychotherapy with a schizophrenic patient and the patient's family.

Ms. Jackson invaded the treatment setting, upsetting other patients, and made the therapist feel anxious, helpless, and angry. She took the therapist's journals, which evoked further feelings of invasion and anger. She provoked disgust with her slovenly appearance. She lied about her attendance at the farm training program, and spent hour upon hour wandering around in the town park. Her uncle grew increasingly unwilling to provide transportation, and the patient understandably felt torn between her own interests and her family's reactions.

In order for this treatment to have had a better chance of success, I think the therapist's interventions should have gone beyond limit setting within the sessions. The following steps should have been taken:

1. The patient should have been referred to a day treatment or vocational setting for a minimum of five days per week. The patient's participation in this program should have been monitored more closely, and noncompliance should have been considered a direct attack on the integrity of the treatment. Too much unstructured time permitted this patient too great an opportunity for unproductive fantasizing and acting out. Such unstructured time can be experienced as an abandonment, and can increase the patient's fears of disorganization and subsequent anxiety and rage. It also can contribute to the patient's denial of his needs for others, and his interpersonal problems by means of autistic withdrawal. In this kind of emotional climate, psychotherapy often carries little weight compared to the patient's fantasies. Moreover, if the patient's social, rehabilitation, medication, and vocational needs are not addressed elsewhere, the psychotherapy is overwhelmed, and cannot focus on the goal for which it is best

suited: to help the patient understand himself psychologically. Two or three sessions per week of psychotherapy cannot replace the whole range of essential treatments needed to help alter a patient's actual life situation. It is fanciful to think that psychotherapy on its own can transform the life circumstances of a patient such as this. At its best, it is a part of an overall approach that includes significant social and vocational rehabilitation. Psychotherapy is a commentary on life, which can lead to changes in affect, attitude, and motivation. But it cannot substitute for learning actual intellectual, social, and vocational skills that the patient needs to master. Such deficiencies, even if they have resulted from psychic conflict, must be met with skilled remediation from tutors, occupational therapists, and vocational counselors.

2. The patient's uncle and aunt should have been included more in the setting up of the treatment. While the plan of the treatment, including the treatment method and the farm program were explained to the Tafts, they did little to monitor the patient's compliance. Both the uncle and aunt were preoccupied with other matters, however, and might not have been able to do this even if it had been stressed.

3. The issue of transportation should have been clarified sooner. Most likely, the uncle's ambivalence about the psychotherapy would have emerged sooner, and the issue could have been discussed more explicitly. The patient might have had more time to integrate the uncle's mixed feelings about the treatment, and discuss it with the therapist.

I would like to emphasize that the outcome of this specific treatment might very well have been the same even if all these issues had been addressed as I have suggested. I use this case to illustrate some of the crucial issues in setting up psychotherapy with schizophrenic patients, not to claim that Ms. Jackson's therapy would necessarily have had a different course.

ENACTMENTS WITHIN THE TREATMENT SETTING

Disruptions in the treatment setting may take rather bizzare forms. Mary Williams was a 20-year-old woman who had lived a very isolated life before admission. She began psychotherapy with

Dr. C, a woman, soon after her hospitalization. During one of the early sessions, the patient wandered around Dr. C's office, trying to unplug all the electrical devices. She tried to take coins from Dr. C's coat, and asked if she could have various articles of clothing. She lay down on the sofa, putting her feet on a nearby chair. On several occasions, she barged into the offices of colleagues in the therapist's suite and would not leave when asked. She constantly tried to put on Dr. C's overcoat, and all Dr. C's efforts at confrontation and interpretation did not help Ms. Williams understand or stop her behavior.

After several weeks of this, the therapist finally told the patient that it would be necessary to meet with her in the living area of the unit, where staff members could observe them. Dr. C said that the staff would help her to be in control so as not to destroy the sessions. The staff would also prevent her from invading Dr. C's privacy. Despite bitter complaints, the patient did attend these sessions, and settled down dramatically. She began to do introspective work for the first time. Dr. C believed that she was reassured that she did not possess the power to blackmail and intimidate the therapist, and thereby destroy the foundations of a serious psychotherapy.

Later on, the patient took to turning her chair so that her back faced the therapist, while affecting a flippant nonchalance about what the therapist was trying to point out to her. Dr. C finally asked the staff members to turn her around. She was shocked and initially outraged that Dr. C would do such a thing, but returned to later sessions more serious and ready to work.

While it is generally not possible in outpatient settings to compel the patient's attendance, or to have colleagues prevent physical disruption, still this case illustrates the need not to accept an unproductive stalemate in the treatment. The patient may feel nihilistic and hopeless, but the therapist should not be overwhelmed by the same feelings of impotence and despair. It is the therapist's responsibility to find creative ways to arrange the conditions for psychotherapy and so begin a collaboration with the patient, or to tell the patient that psychotherapy is not possible. To avoid this is to collude with the part of the patient that wants to destroy meaningful treatment or avoid it altogether. It is to acknowledge tacitly that one is not only impotent but unwilling to face therapeutic reality. This can undermine the patient's residual capacity for reality testing.

Frequently, schizophrenic patients place their therapist in painful dilemmas. On the one hand one does not want to enter into battles with the patient, challenging deeply held beliefs or delusions, running headlong into painful emotional wounds, or provoking rage that can annihilate the relationship. At the same time it is futile to accept a relationship that gratifies the patient's destructiveness, undermines his capacity to separate fantasy from reality, or makes the therapist so uncomfortable that real psychological exploration is impossible. To some it may appear callous to reject a patient because he or she is unwilling to take medication or meet twice a week, or participate in a day hospital program. After all, are these problems not part of the patient's illness? But not to stand by these measures, if they are prerequisites for productive psychotherapy, is not to do the patient any favor. Many patients are used to parental figures who choose expedient, but ultimately unhelpful solutions to grave problems. Many also understand when their efforts to destroy help have succeeded, and they feel abandoned and frightened when they are able to annihilate their treatment.

Moreover, I am not suggesting that all schizophrenic patients must choose to participate in psychotherapy, and that all therapists should refuse to work with them if they do not abide by the necessary preconditions. For some patients, other forms of treatment such as medication, directive treatments, or different forms of psychotherapy may be more acceptable and more useful. But if patient and therapist agree that psychodynamic psychotherapy, with all its potential risks and benefits, should be tried, it does not serve the patient to agree to a treatment structure that cannot succeed.

In emphasizing the importance of prerequisite conditions for beginning psychotherapy, I am not minimizing the patient's impairments, and how difficult it may be to meet such conditions. Dr. V worked with a man for a number of years. It was unclear to him whether this man's diagnosis was paranoid character (DSM-III-R) or whether he was structurally psychotic (Kernberg, 1975, 1984). When confronted about his paranoid beliefs, the patient consistently became evasive and more agitated. Nevertheless, he maintained a senior administrative position in a university, and had some friends and several girl friends. These relationships were essentially need satisfying and shallow. His sister, and probably his uncle, were schizophrenic. It was difficult for the patient to empathize with others, and disappointment led not only to his seeing others as all bad, but to severe paranoid anxieties. His predominant defenses were splitting, projective identification, omnipotent control, and denial.

On one occasion the patient expressed suicidal ideas and agreed to a contract. He would not harm himself, but would call the therapist every day or two; however, on several occasions, he did not. Moreover, when the therapist called there was no answer. This left Dr. V feeling quite anxious, having little information upon which to make the decision whether to call the patient's relatives to find out if he was safe. The patient later told Dr. V that he had "fallen asleep" and so could not call. The therapist emphasized that it was essential at times of crisis that he be able to contact the patient reliably, otherwise the therapist would be unable to be calm enough to listen to the patient in sessions, and they would not be able to work together.

Several months later, the patient became more and more paranoid. His suspicions did not diminish with confrontation and interpretation. He went on to develop a transference psychosis. He came to a session with only ten minutes left, and then talked distractedly about seemingly trivial details of the day. During the next session he reported some suicidal thoughts, and agreed to make a brief office visit the next day to see Dr. V for follow-up. Dr. V waited, but the patient never came. Dr. V received no phone call or message. Finally, he called the patient's office. The patient, he learned, had gone to an academic meeting out of town. Upon the patient's return, Dr. V discontinued the psychotherapy, referred the patient elsewhere, and explained that he had destroyed conditions necessary for Dr. V to work with him. Dr. V said that because of the patient's lack of contact, he was constantly worried about the patient's safety, and this made it impossible for him to think calmly and clearly about the patient's psychotherapy.

It was difficult for Dr. V to terminate this treatment. Both the patient and the therapist had put in time and effort. But Dr. V felt that if the treatment had continued, there would be no effective limit on the patient's use of suicidal threats as sadistic gratifications, and as self-destructive attempts to destroy the psychotherapy. In addition, during the periods in which the patient was incommunicado, Dr. V found himself so preoccupied with the concrete details of the patient's whereabouts and safety, that he really did not have the psychological "space" to reflect on his dynamics and defenses and to formulate a good understanding of what was going on. Dr. V also found himself so preoccupied with countertransference fear, worry, anger, and resentment that it was difficult for him to think creatively. Perhaps the patient could use his experience of destroying this treatment to pause, reflect, and begin another psychotherapy in a more constructive way.

Mr. Green had been seeing Dr. H for about one year when he started to work at a paying job. He used much of this money to buy expensive sports and electronic equipment. Up to this time his family had been paying for his treatment. About six months after he started at his job, Dr. H began to discuss the possibility of his contributing to the payment. He became furious, accused Dr. H of being "money hungry," and protested that he could not part with any of his money. He became extremely suspicious and combative, saying that Dr. H did not want him to get better. In fact, he declared, he would not discuss this subject any more.

Dr. H felt that it was important for this patient to pay something because he had devalued the treatment in many overt and covert ways. He had skipped appointments to go skiing, and rarely paid on time. Now, he seemed to be saying that the therapy might be worth his *parents'* money, but not his own hard-earned savings.

After some time the patient agreed to pay. His participation in his treatment became noticeably more serious and productive. Not paying had been a way of expressing derogation of Dr. H, of maintaining an image of himself as both infantile and special, and of holding onto a self-destructive attachment to his parents whom he felt were engulfing and undermining.

Some enactments are subtle and operate via their countertransference impact on the therapist. I will discuss this further in chapter 4, but will give an example here. Mr. DeVito had been in treatment for many years. There had been ups and downs, but he had remained out of the hospital for five years and was functioning at work. Nevertheless, the sessions had taken on a repetitive, dull, and soporific quality for months. The patient had gained weight, he dressed drably, and had little to talk about in the meetings. He really seemed like a formless lump. In response, the therapist's mind wandered, and at times, during the long silences, he fell into a kind of distracted reverie. He felt comfortable and snug, as if he had just been put into a cozy bed by a parent. At times, he really did not want to be disturbed out of his cozy corner, and have to "wake up" to conduct psychotherapy. After the therapist realized what was going on, he discussed his reactions with Mr. DeVito, and both were able to see that the therapist's feelings mirrored those of the patient.

I will discuss in chapters 4 and 5 how this countertransference issue can be handled. I offer this example here to illustrate how subtle enactments by the patient can have an important impact on the therapist.

ENACTMENTS OUTSIDE THE THERAPY

The behavior of patients outside the consulting room can also have an important effect on their treatments. Ronald White was a 20-year-old British man with a borderline personality and psychotic depression.[1] He came for treatment because of a depressive episode, but decided to work in psychotherapy on his social isolation. After a few months, it emerged that he was taking items from the warehouse where he worked and reselling them for cash. When Dr. W asked about this, Mr. White replied that all the guys at work did this, and, moreover, that unless he stole these things, he could not afford the treatment. Earlier on in treatment, Mr. White had expressed skepticism about the genuineness of the therapist's interest. He was interested, Mr. White contended, because he got paid.

After several weeks' discussion the stealing had not abated. Finally, Dr. W told the patient that he would not continue to see him if he stole. His stealing represented a deep cynicism about relationships, including the one with Dr. W. It reflected a belief that he could not get something valuable from someone else by their freely giving it—he had to take it against their will, or without their knowledge. And more importantly, in the context of the therapy, it gratified the anger implicit in his hostile image of

---

[1]Despite Mr. White's diagnosis of affective disorder, this is a good example of aspects of work with schizophrenic patients as well.

Dr. W. He essentially saw Dr. W as a hypocrite who professed ethical values, but who did not really care if he was paid with profits from stolen goods, as long as he got paid. Eventually, Mr. White agreed to stop stealing, and was able to explore many of these issues.

Many enactments may not appear to be enactments at all, but just part of the patient's illness. After five years out of the hospital Mr. DeVito made tentative efforts to establish a relationship with a woman, and move out from his aunt and uncle's home. Finally, he did move out and talked with his girl friend about marriage. Within six months he was hospitalized five times. At least two or three of his previous hospitalizations were associated with his moving away from his relatives to live independently. Mr. DeVito's symptoms were florid; he had auditory hallucinations and paranoid delusions. On an impulse, he drove his motorcycle to California where he was picked up by the police for vagrancy. With all this, Dr. B, his therapist, felt that the patient made use of his symptoms to avoid the emotional stresses related to intimacy and separation. Moreover, with each hospitalization, Mr. DeVito lost his job and was forced to depend even more heavily on his aunt and uncle. At one point, he spent many months out of work, waking up late and going to the racetrack. He acted, actually, as if he were a man of independent means, living a rather carefree, if limited, existence. There was a bland and thoroughgoing denial of the real life consequences of the impact of all this on his work and personal life.

While Dr. B understood that the patient had a psychotic disorder, nevertheless he felt that the frequency of the recent hospitalizations, and the nature of his posthospital adjustment were enactments, and that the patient was capable of greater control. Dr. B and the patient discussed these issues in treatment, and developed a plan. They agreed that if the patient were hospitalized again, that within four weeks he would be working at a paying job that could support his treatment, or the psychotherapy would be suspended until such time that the patient was earning an income.[2] The purpose of this plan was to help reduce Mr. DeVito's denial of the destructive impact of his hospitalizations

---

[2]Under these circumstances, Dr. B would continue to prescribe medication and would be available in emergencies. The patient would follow up with any aftercare rehabilitation program that had been set up in the hospital.

on his capacity to function as an adult. Another goal was to reduce the patient's effort to turn the psychotherapy into a kind of compensation for past suffering paid for by his uncle which he would then take pleasure in destroying.

Sometimes, schizophrenic patients do not destroy treatment by gratifying primitive impulses or by destroying the therapist's equanimity, but by undermining the social or financial support necessary to keep the treatment going. The case of Helen Jackson provides a good example. The patient's uncle was providing transportation to the treatment. One of the family's unstated objectives was that Ms. Jackson not interfere with their everyday lives. For her part, the patient was enraged about what she felt to be past and current abandonments. Her throwing garbage out of the window expressed considerable anger toward her aunt and uncle. Although the patient and Dr. S discussed the impact of these acts, and the fragile nature of her uncle's support, she persisted. Whether she wanted to sabotage her treatment by undermining the support of the Tafts, or whether there was another motive, she did succeed in making her family progressively more exasperated and finally desperate, it seemed, to find some treatment that would contain her. Her uncle finally told her to stop coming to sessions.

Ms. Chen had been in treatment for four years. She had, for the first time, established a relationship with a man over an extended period of time. They spent long weekends together. This was quite a strain at times for the patient, who scrupulously tried to maintain her "personal space." She was extremely sensitive to perceived slights, and reacted with explosive anger. When her boyfriend criticized her for forgetting to buy concert tickets, she exploded in fury, abandoning him, her job, and her psychotherapy. She maintained sporadic contact with her therapist after that, but remained out of work for many months. Even if she had wanted to return to psychotherapy, she could not have done so because she could not have afforded it. In her fury, she had not only burned interpersonal bridges, but financial ones as well.

Of course, there is no limit to the variety of enactments which can jeopardize the psychotherapy of schizophrenic patients. One cannot coercively suppress all unusual, idiosyncratic, imprudent, or pathologically gratifying impulses. The goal of psychotherapy is change via self-understanding and integration, not compliance or submission to the psychiatrist's image of normality or ideal health. At the same time, while recognizing the danger of excessive control, patients can act in ways that severely compromise the possibility of verbal psychotherapy. It is the therapist's job to evaluate how much the treatment may be compromised and to weigh the comparative value of setting a limit. At times, some of the limits one sets may appear controlling or callous to an outside observer, including members of the patient's family. As much as possible these limits should be explained to both the patient and family.

There are no simple rules of thumb in deciding when and how to set a limit, and these strategic clinical judgments may be quite subtle and complicated. It should be stressed that in making such difficult decisions about limits, the therapist will inevitably make mistakes, not going far enough in some instances, and going too far in others. Nevertheless, it is no favor to the patient to avoid thinking them through, and, if necessary, introducing them. In the end, one may be able to discuss the need for having set limits with the patient, and eventually eliminate them. This is not possible if the patient has already dropped out, or if the patient and therapist have entered a chronic and unproductive stalemate.

I will end this chapter by listing below a set of conditions for effective psychotherapy with a schizophrenic patient. The list is obviously incomplete, and is intended to be illustrative and not a prescription for any individual case.

1. Willingness to take medication.
2. Willingness to participate in a full-time, five-day per week constructive activity such as work, a day hospital program, or rehabilitation.
3. Willingness to pay, or find and preserve financial support.
4. Willingness to refrain from attacks or intrusions on the physical setting of the treatment or the therapist.
5. As in work with borderline patients, willingness to report feelings or actions which may lead to danger to the patient or others.

Chapter 4

The Psychological Therapy of Schizophrenic Patients

THE NATURE OF PSYCHIC STRUCTURE IN SCHIZOPHRENIA

The goal of medical treatment is either the removal or arrest of the underlying disease processes which lead to symptoms. If this is not possible, treatment aims at reducing symptoms, and increasing or at least preserving function. This is no less true for psychoanalytic therapy. With neurotic patients, we are used to goals which are extremely ambitious: the reduction of psychic conflicts which cause symptoms and character disorder. Certain writers (Rosen, 1953; Boyer and Giovachini, 1967, 1980; Rosenfeld, 1969) believe that we do not need to reduce or dilute these goals when we work with schizophrenic patients. Others (e.g., Federn, 1943a,b,c) have suggested more modest ambitions, focusing on symptom reduction. They hold that it is not possible to reorganize pathological structure.

The psychotherapy techniques I will describe do not presume that this debate need be resolved. It remains for us to discover how far such techniques can go in reducing symptoms or reorganizing psychic structure. They are designed to address five areas of psychopathology which have been considered crucial in understanding the psychology of schizophrenia, namely:

1. The disturbance in the capacity for emotional attachment;
2. The disturbance in affect awareness and regulation;
3. The disturbance in the development and preservation of psychological boundaries;

4. The disturbance in symbol use;
5. The disturbance in the testing of reality.

These techniques aim not only at fostering useful social habits (Liberman, Lillie, Falloon, Harpin, Hutchinson, and Stoute, 1984; Liberman, Massel, Most, and Wong, 1985; Liberman, Mueser, and Wallace, 1986) as helpful as this may be, but also attempt at another level to have an impact on underlying psychopathology. As I discussed in the Introduction, my working hypothesis is that psychotic psychopathology *may* have important roots in psychological conflict, and that it is important to design techniques to address the psychological pathology of schizophrenia, such as the five areas of disturbance noted above.

Whatever the ultimate goal of treatment, effective psychological therapy will call upon the patient's capacity for verbal symbol use and concept formation. In discussing psychoanalysis as a talking cure, Freud (1916–1917) addressed the criticism that the treatment was "only words" and therefore somehow gossamer. He emphasized the power of words, and their influence as agents of change. He went so far as to say that the goal of psychoanalytic treatment was to reproduce the patient's pathological impressions in words, and "the therapeutic task *consists solely* in inducing him to do so" (Breuer and Freud, 1895, p. 283). Whether the long-range objectives for the psychological treatment of the schizophrenic patient are symptom reduction or psychic reorganization, the immediate goal must always be to help the patient put his experience into words. Since effective treatment usually requires a long period of time, and since overall success depends so completely on the use of words, this immediate goal, at least at the outset, becomes the *fundamental practical goal*. None of the other therapeutic aims of a verbal psychotherapy, such as affect tolerance, control of impulses, or self-understanding, can occur if the patient cannot succeed in putting his experience into appropriate words. This is a necessary, although not sufficient, condition for progress in verbal psychotherapy. Without it, treatment can only consist of changes brought about by medicine, or changes in behavior caused by manipulative treatments such as operant conditioning, punishment, and so on. Thus, in many cases where symptomatic change may be very slow, psychotherapy must address a provisional and more immediate goal: helping the patient to use words.

PSYCHIC STRUCTURE AND THE DISTURBANCES OF EGO FUNCTIONING

Before discussing psychotherapy techniques which are useful in working with schizophrenic patients, it is important to identify the ways in which the psychic structure of schizophrenic patients differs from that of neurotics. The structural disturbances proceed from modifications or impairments in the patient's ego functioning. If, for example, the schizophrenic has difficulty using words and symbols (Goldstein, 1944), then a standard, strictly verbal form of treatment, based exclusively on interpretation, will not succeed. As noted above, there are five broad areas of ego pathology which stand out in schizophrenia, each of which has been described by a number of psychoanalytic writers. These enduring "modifications" (Eissler, 1953a) in the way the ego functions, I believe, constitute a characteristic psychic structure which differs both from that found in neurosis and borderline conditions.

Disturbance in the Capacity for Emotional Attachment

Many analytic authors have written about the brittleness and vulnerability of the schizophrenic's object attachments (Freud, 1911, 1914, 1924a,b; Fenichel, 1945; Hartmann, 1953). Schizophrenic patients make human connections with great caution. It is as if a great barrier must be overcome. Despite intense affect, these connections are vulnerable to being broken off abruptly with little provocation, and little warning. These attachments do not have the "staying power" to withstand disappointment, loss, or rage. They can quickly change from having a positive emotional tone, to having a paranoid one (see Sullivan's concept of "malignant transformation" [Sullivan, 1962]).

   Early on, it had been thought (Freud, 1916–1917; Fenichel, 1945) that schizophrenic patients were unable to develop a transference neurosis. Later, clinicians came to believe (Fromm-Reichmann, 1959; Searles, 1965, 1979; Sullivan, 1962) that it was not the *absence* of attachment or transference that characterized schizophrenia, but its *quality*. Of the patients described in this book, Ms. Chen stands out as a fitting example. She established a suspicious but very intense attachment both to her therapist, and to her boyfriend. This connection could withstand only modest disappointments and disruptions, but not more. When the patient's boyfriend made a comment the patient perceived as too critical, she reacted with violent rage, ending the relationship with boyfriend, employer, and therapist in a paranoid fury.

Disturbance in Affect Awareness and Regulation

Many writers have observed that schizophrenics have difficulty containing, toning down, and integrating their impulses, especially aggressive ones (Hartmann, 1953; Bak, 1954); these may break through unmodified. The patient may become verbally abusive, physically threatening, or provocative. Recall Ms. Chen's explosions of anger, and Ms. Williams' intrusive antics in the office. Ms. Weiss felt driven to kill her boss and others who offended her. When Mr. DeVito became psychotic, all kinds of sexual and aggressive impulses burst forth.

Patients may try to escape from the danger of their impulses by becoming excessively passive, even stuporous or emotionally withdrawn. Or, they may project their hostile impulses onto others. Ms. Williams reported late in her inpatient treatment that in the early sessions, she had felt like jumping up and choking Dr. C. At the same time, she was afraid that Dr. C. would kill her.

Hartmann (1953) believed that the schizophrenic's inability to "neutralize" aggression undermined the development of normal countercathexes. This made repression impossible. Thus, he connected the ego's difficulty in mastering aggression with a disturbance of the normal boundary between the ego and the id.

Disturbance in the Development and Preservation of Psychological Boundaries

The schizophrenic patient not only shows a disturbance in the boundary between the ego and the id (Federn, 1943a,b,c; Hartmann, 1953), but also between the ego and the outside world.

One of the cardinal and most consequential disturbances in schizophrenia is the patient's difficulty in discriminating what is inside and what is outside, and what is self and what is other. The capacity to distinguish inner from outer experience, what I will call the "sense of boundary," is central to differentiating between perceptions, feelings, memories, fantasies, and thoughts, and thus is central to the capacity to test inner (Hartmann, 1953), as well as external reality (Kernberg, 1975).[1] A disturbance of the sense of boundary is intimately linked to such defenses as primitive projection, psychotic identification, fusion of self and object images, and animation and deanimation (Mahler, 1968), and, consequently, such psychotic symptoms as paranoid ideas, ideas of reference, and gross disturbances of identity. It is not clear how a disturbance in the sense of boundary arises; whether it is a disturbance in a normal developmental phase, a product of pathological processes such as primitive defense, or involves psychobiological factors such as a defect in a stimulus barrier.

Ms. Williams reported late in her hospital stay that she feared Dr. C would attack her, and that this coincided with her own impulses to stand up and punch her therapist. She was unable to discern who wanted to murder whom. Mr. DeVito heard voices outside his head accusing him of being a gangster. When he was not psychotic, he had repeatedly complained that his aunt had mistreated and abused him. Apparently, when he was psychotic, it was no longer clear who was the abuser and who the abused. At work, Ms. Chen repeatedly left cryptic messages in the staff mailboxes, in which she made obscure observations about her colleagues. When her symptoms became worse, she believed that it was her colleagues who were cryptically communicating with her by leaving paper cups in certain patterns near the water cooler, and by wearing outfits with special colors. A man who was acutely psychotic came to the emergency room and claimed that he was Ted Koppel, J. Edgar Hoover, and Bart Simpson all in one. Clearly, his sense of identity was neither well defined nor even unitary.

---

[1] I hesitate to refer to this boundary phenomenon as a boundary *function* because I do not want to imply that there is a unitary function of the ego whose role it is to formulate a distinct ego boundary. I also do not want to imply that the sense of such a boundary develops or is disturbed only on a psychological basis.

In terms of object relations, a disturbance in the sense of boundary leads the patient to feel helplessly at the mercy of affects stirred up by another person. The patient feels that there is nothing to shield him from powerful longings, disappointments, excitements, and losses stirred up by the object's behavior. The patient feels buffeted by these external stimuli, that he is out of control, and often, that his inner life is being controlled or manipulated by the object. These experiences contribute to the patient's sense of vulnerability to pain initiated by the outside world, and lays the groundwork for organizing experience in a paranoid way. They also have a powerful impact on self-esteem. Patients feel unable to stem feelings of helplessness, shame, and impotence. Some patients defensively distance themselves from objects, making use of paranoid fantasies to justify their isolation. Eventually, for some, this isolation serves only to increase their feeling of loss and disconnectedness. In time, the hunger for contact leads to renewed and more desperate needs for the object, and new and more intense fears of engulfment begin (see chapters 5 and 6 on the disturbance in the sense of boundary and its relation to paranoia).

During her psychotherapy, Ms. Chen felt alternately close to and distant from her therapist. When her therapist made a transference interpretation that hit home, Ms. Chen's feeling understood was often accompanied by a feeling of being under that therapist's control. At these times, she had the bodily sensation that her therapist was grasping her ear with metal pincers. At other times, when she felt her therapist was too close to her, she had the sensation of feeling somehow shriveled and smaller, as if her skin were loose like a deflated balloon. Such experiences led her continually to try to reestablish a distance by canceling sessions, or by perceiving the therapist as an adversary.

The blurring of the boundary between self and other has been emphasized by many authors (Freud, 1914, 1921, 1923, 1925; Fenichel, 1945; A. Reich, 1954; Greenacre, 1958; Mahler, 1958, 1963, 1968; Lampl-de Groot, 1962; Jacobson, 1964; Greenson, 1968; Stoller, 1974; Kernberg, 1975; Person and Ovesey, 1978; Bergman, 1982). This boundary disturbance may arise in different ways. The patients who experience their affects or self representations as intolerable, may want to believe that it is the therapist who possesses all their unacceptable parts, and may use primitive defenses (e.g., projective identification or primitive denial) to attempt to force these parts, in fantasy, into the therapist (Klein, 1946; Kernberg, 1975). As a result, the boundary between self and other may become confused. Or, the patient may seek regressive refusion of self and object images (Jacobson, 1964, 1967) in an effort to establish a safe, stable object relationship that is insured, so to speak, against change and loss. This effort, obviously, can contribute to boundary confusion. Of course, it may be that developmentally, the patient may never have achieved an adequate psychic separation from the object (Mahler, 1968; Loewald, 1980) (another mechanism for the blurring of the selfobject boundary is suggested in chapter 6). In any event, the tendency to confuse self and object images is a crucial factor in the development of psychotic symptomatology.

Disturbance in Symbol Use

The schizophrenic patient shows a disturbance in his use of symbols in general, and language in particular. Freud (1915) explained this by postulating a division between the "thing" presentation and the "word" (or verbal) presentation of an object. He believed that in schizophrenia, the two became uncoupled and the patient clings to the "word" presentation to find his way back to the external reality which he has lost. Many other writers have described and theorized about the alternating concreteness and abstractness of schizophrenic speech (Klein, 1923, 1930).

One facet of the disturbance in symbol use is the apparent loss of the capacity for concept formation (abstraction) and, as a consequence, of much of the experience of meaning. Where once concepts and meanings existed, and importantly, the affects which accompanied them (Searles, 1979, p. 16), new sensations and perceptions seem to spring up. There appears to be a kind of desymbolizing (Searles, 1965), or, more specifically, a deconceptualizing of experience. In its stead, the patient seems to be beset by all kinds of uncanny and bizarre somatic, perceptual, and sensory experiences. One might speculate that the evolution of conceptual thought from concrete sensation has been reversed (see chapter 6).

When Mr. DeVito first described what he later identified as sadness, he said that he could literally feel his heart in his chest. He said it was sliding down because it "weighs so much." When Ms. Chen was criticized by her school principal, she did not report feeling that her sense of identity was threatened, but instead had the physical sensation that her "body had shrunk" and was now "small and painful." The same patient, as noted above, experienced her skin as "loose and shriveled" when she felt that her therapist has disparaged her. She was not conscious of feeling painfully vulnerable to being hurt by her doctor, or that the doctor had betrayed her budding affection by deflating her sense of her own value, or any other emotion which would have fit the emotional context.

On the other side, certain schizophrenic patients are given to conceptual vagueness and obfuscation. For these individuals, as Freud noted in his discussion of "Words and Things" (1915, pp. 209–215), words seem to have lost their moorings, and no longer reliably designate an agreed-upon referent. They are like buoys which have broken loose, wandering about in the sea, no longer marking reliable locations in any systematic way. One feels one has lost one's way among vague, stilted, and scattered verbal signs. Occasionally, this has been referred to as "overabstraction," but this kind of mental activity is not really abstraction in that no true concept formation (Vygotsky, 1934; Piaget and Inhelder, 1969) or class-concept use (Langer, 1967) is taking place.

Instead, such verbal productions may be intended more to obscure communication than to advance it. Speech serves to hide as well as to communicate, as Orwell's famous examples in *Nineteen Eighty-Four* (1949) show. Ms. Williams said as much when she talked about her incoherent orations at activities therapy. In a moment of candor she explained "When I talk that way in activities therapy it's so no one will know what feelings I'm really having."

If, in fact, symbol use is defective in schizophrenia, then a psychotherapy which depends primarily on interpretation of symbolic expressions, by means of symbols, and which presumes an already well-functioning "symbolic apparatus," is compromised from the beginning. Searles (1979) has written, "A patient who is experiencing himself as a shifting flux of somatic sensations, thoughts, mental images, memories and so on, is in no condition to hear or utilize a verbal interpretation from the analyst'' (p. 145). It would seem that the first order of business in psychotherapy with schizophrenic patients would be to address the defect in symbol use. Without some improvement in this ego function, the traditional analytic tools of clarification, confrontation, and interpretation are robbed of their power.

DISTURBANCE IN THE TESTING OF REALITY

The breakdown of the capacity to test reality has been identified by most writers as the defining disturbance in psychosis (Freud, 1924a,b; Fenichel, 1945; Kernberg, 1975, 1984). For Kernberg, this ego function consists of the capacity to discriminate internal from external sources of perception, the capacity to differentiate self from object, and the capacity to empathize with the social criteria of reality (1975, 1984). What I would like to add to these formulations is that these ego capacities in turn rest upon the integrity of the ego's ability to use concepts. If symbols and concepts become degraded into their perceptual and sensational building blocks,[1] then the door is opened to confusion about the source of phenomenal experience. Similarly, if the experience of interpersonal influence is deconceptualized and perceptualized, this may lead to the concrete perception of a lack of boundary between self and object. Finally, if the world of conceptual thought is lost, the individual loses, pari passu, his link to the world of shared cultural meaning. Thus, his empathy with the social criteria of reality is lost. The mechanisms by which deconceptualization and desymbolization may compromise reality testing are discussed further in chapter 6.

The list of ego disturbances discussed above is by no means comprehensive. Its does however, designate a set of dysfunctions which have been identified by a large number of writers from diverse theoretical backgrounds. These disorders may be said to comprise a ''core'' of ego psychopathology about which some consensus has developed. A psychotherapy of schizophrenia should take into account the pathology of the ego in these areas.

---

[1]See discussion in chapter 6, particularly pp. 180–182.

It must combine a rational plan to ameliorate them, as well as an appreciation of how the basic model technique of psychoanalysis must be modified in order to work within the limits imposed by these ego modifications.

PSYCHOTHERAPY TECHNIQUES

General Principles

Before describing individual techniques for psychotherapy with schizophrenics, I would like to emphasize some general principles of technique which are important to keep in mind regardless of one's specific intervention.

Monitoring the Interpersonal Relationship

It would lead us too far from the central discussion to examine here the question of whether a "real" relationship (Greenson, 1967) exists between a patient and his therapist that is distinct from the transference. Similarly, whether patients are capable of developing a "new" transference, or only repeat infantile experiences, cannot be taken up at length. My own perspective is that it is useful to draw a distinction between the transference and the "interpersonal relationship" between patient and therapist in work with schizophrenic patients.

First, the distortion of the image of the therapist is not limited to transference of the neurotic type. It depends also on massive disruptions in ego functioning, some of which are caused by primitive defensive operations such as projective identification, primitive denial, and fusion of self and object images. The therapist is not routinely perceived only as a new edition of an actual past object, but often as a figure which is grossly distorted by past and present defenses and failures in ego function (Kernberg, 1975). What might be a question of a dynamically motivated substitution of past for present in a neurotic (within the bounds of good reality testing) becomes, in the schizophrenic, a frank break with reality. With neurotics, patient and therapist can agree that a certain feeling or thought does not rationally "fit" in the present relationship with the therapist, and must therefore represent the effect of an emotion based in the past. With the schizophrenic, there is often no such shared, detached viewpoint. In the patient's view, he does not *imagine* that the therapist is dishonest, persecutory, uncaring, controlling or malicious; the therapist *is* these things. If the schizophrenic patient does not agree that a certain emotion is based in transference, one cannot interpret it to him as such. In my own mind, I find it useful to think of such experiences as "interactional" or "interpersonal." I leave the clarification of transference phenomena for later exploration, when the patient is more able to appreciate how his perceptions may be distorted. For the present, I focus on how the patient's beliefs arise from the evidence he has gathered, how these beliefs or this evidence fit with what else he knows, and whether his conclusions develop logically from this information. Helping the patient with his testing of reality proceeds pari passu with this approach. This way of working often involves reviewing, examining, and explaining the therapist's view of the interaction with the patient, steps not necessary with patients whose reality testing is intact.

In work with neurotic patients one might say there is a "neutral" area in which both patient and therapist understand the following: that a doctor–patient relationship has been established, that it involves certain practical financial and schedule arrangements, that patient and therapist have different and well-delineated roles, that they will have little if any social contact, and that the therapist's role is not to become a gratifying figure in the patient's life. This neutral area is often invaded and under siege in work with schizophrenics. Ms. Williams and Ms. Jackson barged in on sessions with other patients. Both rummaged through personal belongings in the therapist's office. Patients may try to follow the therapist from his office, or call him at his home, or refuse to leave the consulting room. No doubt, these behaviors are connected to infantile transferences. But the boundary between what is the patient and what is the therapist has been so abridged, the capacity to empathize with the therapist's role so compromised, the use of primitive defense and the operation of pathological ego functions so widespread, that it is hard to conceptualize these behaviors as straightforward repetitions or faithful replicas of developmental experience. Moreover, it is usually futile therapeutically to link such behaviors with past experience. Since the patient does not acknowledge that his own distortions based on the past may be playing a role in his relation to the therapist, I find it useful to think of these experiences as "interactional," focusing on the here-and-now.

Finally, I would like to make what may be an obvious point. Work with schizophrenic patients often involves more activity and actual self-revelation on the part of the therapist than with neurotic or borderline patients. One can reasonably assume then that at least some of the patient's reactions to the therapist occur in response to emotions and ideas which the therapist expresses, and actions which he takes.

One of the major causes for failure in psychotherapy with schizophrenic patients is the inability to establish a working relationship. The patient flees from treatment because of real or imagined qualities of the therapist. Introspection and self-disclosure will never occur without some rudimentary belief in the therapist's honesty, dependability, and self-control. The therapeutic alliance or "pact" (Freud, 1940) depends on such a groundwork, and everything which might interfere with it should be carefully monitored. The patient, for example, may be offended by the therapist's mood or tone. He may be angry about a rescheduled meeting, or the denial of a request. The therapist must ask himself constantly: what kind of relationship do I have with the patient now? Does he feel spiteful? Is he envious? Does he feel hurt? What behavior of mine might have triggered these feelings, or might intensify them? How will these feelings influence the patient's willingness to put his thoughts and feelings into words?

Monitoring the Transference

What I have said above does not mean that the therapist should not be alert to the repetition of past object relations in the present. All phenomena, verbal and behavioral, in and out of sessions, must be considered in the light of their relationship to the therapist and their historical meanings. For schizophrenic patients, whose lives are often empty interpersonally and intrapsychically, the relationship with the therapist can assume enormous importance. Negative transferences based on past object relations can have a particularly destructive impact on the treatment alliance.

Ms. Chen, the middle-aged teacher, was extremely concerned that greater closeness meant that the therapist would manipulate her. It was very important to her sense of psychological integrity that she maintain her "personal space." One could well understand her concern in terms of her impaired sense of boundary, her wishes for and fears of fusion, and her use of primitive projection. Nevertheless, it was also the case that Ms. Chen's mother had been shockingly intrusive during her childhood. Despite her daughter's passion for swimming, her mother pressured her to discontinue participation in after-school athletic activities. She repeatedly gave heavy-handed direction about her studies and friendships. She even called the parents of her daughter's friends to push her daughter in what she felt was the right direction.

Monitoring the Countertransference

A variety of authors, with different theoretical points of view, have observed that countertransference reactions can provide essential information about the subjective state of the patient. As used in this sense, the term *countertransference* refers not to the therapist's idiosyncratic image of the patient as a current version of an object from his own past, but rather to the thoughts, feelings, and impulses which occur to him as he responds to what the patient says or does. Arlow (1980) has written about such reactions in psychoanalysis: "No matter how distant the context of his thoughts may seem from the patient's preoccupations, he (the analyst) nevertheless appreciates them as clues or signals pointing to the unconscious meaning of the patient's communications" (p. 204).

If attention to this phenomenon is important in work with neurotics, then it is indispensable in work with schizophrenics. Rosenfeld (1954) has written that such countertransference reactions are often the "only guide" to what is happening with a chaotic or uncommunicative patient. Because the patient's capacity for symbolic communication is frequently impaired, voluntary verbal communication may be impossible. The more such commincation breaks down, the more it seems that the patient relies upon inducing emotions and thoughts in the therapist by nonverbal means (Lotterman, 1990), and the more vital it is that the therapist makes use of his own capacity to be a "receiving set" (Freud, 1912; Rosenfeld, 1952) for such signals.

Respect for Psychic Determinism

Freud (1916–1917) emphasized that seemingly bizarre or incomprehensible behavior or mental events had a "sense." This awareness is no less important in working with schizophrenics than it is with neurotics. In fact, it is perhaps more so, because schizophrenic thought and behavior appear so much more "senseless" and so much more difficult to comprehend than that of neurotic patients. Often, schizophrenics cannot even produce sensible rationalizations for their symptomatic behavior as neurotic patients can, adding to the impression of its senselessness. In any case, there is a greater prejudice among clinicians against seeing the sense behind psychotic symptoms, especially when those symptoms cause disruptions in the process of verbal communication. In practice, loose associations are rarely viewed as symptoms with a sense, but rather are seen to be evidence of a neurochemical or neuroanatomic diathesis. Again, I am not attempting to discount the relevance of somatic or genetic factors in schizophrenia. I am saying that even in the case of such dramatic symptoms as looseness of association, concreteness of thought, auditory hallucinations, or paranoid delusions, it is profitable to consider that the patient's acts or thoughts, even though bizarre, may have a sense or may communicate something important. While there is no guarantee that this approach will always bear fruit and will always uncover hidden meanings, such meanings can never be found without the commitment to search for them.

Dorothy Bender, a 40-year-old woman, had a long-standing history of paranoid delusions, auditory hallucinations, social isolation, idiosyncratic and bizarre behavior, and marked disturbances in thinking and speech, but no history or prominent affective symptoms or organic pathology. Her diagnosis was schizophrenia according to DSM-III-R criteria (APA, 1987) and she was psychotic by structural criteria as well. Early in one session, Dr. M asked her what had led to her troubles with her family with whom she had fought a great deal. After fending off this question several times, she said that she saw something blurry and indistinct next to Dr. M's chair. Her therapist asked her about it and she appeared uninterested and otherwise preoccupied. Dr. M decided to persevere, and asked her to describe in as much detail as she could what the object looked like, how big it was, what shape it seemed to have, what the surface appearance was, and so on. She said that it seemed to become more clear and looked like sandpaper. Its surface looked rough and abrasive. "It has the appearance of someone who is irritating and pushy." This opened up a discussion of how irritating and grating it was that Dr. M continued to probe about her family conflicts, which Ms. Bender did not want to discuss. What appeared from one point of view to be an irrelevant and bothersome sensory malfunction, turned out to have a lot of meaning.

Specific Techniques

Parameters

In discussing the psychoanalytic treatment of certain patients Eissler (1953a) suggested that departures from the basic model technique of psychoanalysis might be necessary. He termed such technical departures *parameters* and suggested guidelines for using them. Historically, one purpose of these modifications has been to limit the unproductive acting out of certain patients. Kernberg (1975, 1984) has made the use of such parameters a building block of his technique with severe character disorders. It is outside the scope of this work to discuss whether such parameters represent a departure from psychoanalytic treatment or not. My own view is that they are compatible with psychoanalytic therapy. In any case, the psychotherapy of schizophrenics usually cannot occur without such parameters, at least at some point. Schizophrenic patients, no less than borderline patients, can be impulsive, provocative, and destructive of their treatments. Parameters may consist of rules concerning behavior in and out of the sessions, and they serve several functions. First they can serve to protect the therapist's technical neutrality so that, for example, he does not become too intimidated, or too angry. Second, they prevent the patient from destroying conditions necessary for a successful therapy by such means as self-cutting, manipulative suicide attempts, or attending sessions while intoxicated. Third, they can be designed to limit the gratification rather than the verbal working through of primitive impulses. As I discussed in chapter

3, to refrain from responding to blatant provocation and destruction of the treatment setting by such activities as yelling, touching
the therapist, or destroying property, is to permit the pathology
of the patient to triumph. To listen inertly in such circumstances
is not technical neutrality, but may be closer to denial, reflecting
a fanciful wish that the disorganized or out-of-control patient will,
somehow, on his own, come to his senses.

Theoretically, parameters include any temporary modification of standard psychoanalytic technique which is designed to
assist in the development of a psychoanalytic process. Certainly,
one of the most important parameters is the setting of limits. A
number of examples were given in chapter 3, and will not be
repeated here. However, many of the specific techniques I will
now discuss, such as disclosing induced emotion, self-disclosure
as part of object definition, naming, enlargement, and role-play-
ing, fall into the category of parameters of technique. One may
argue that these techniques do not keep the modification of psychoanalytic therapy to "a bare minimum" (Eissler, 1953a), that
with schizophrenic patients they are used over long periods of
time, and that, in the end, they may not be resolved by interpretation. Nevertheless, they are designed to increase the chance that
a psychoanalytic process will develop, based upon the uncovering
and interpretation of unconscious thoughts and feelings arising
out of the relationship with the therapist. They may also be essential in approaching resistances to psychological therapy which
strictly verbal approaches have not succeeded in addressing. Parameters of technique are designed to facilitate, not replace, the
psychodynamic process. In some cases, when the patient is better
able to identify and report his inner states in words and concepts,
the use of these parameters becomes less imperative.

Object Definition

In the basic model technique of psychoanalysis (Eissler, 1953a),
the analyst remains a relatively dim, poorly defined figure. This
permits regression in the patient and a more rapid, full-blown
transference to develop. While neurotic patients with intact reality
testing can make creative and adaptive use of this regression as
a source of information about themselves, borderline patients
often cannot do so, and are vulnerable to confusing transference

and reality; that is to say, they may experience a transference psychosis (Rosenfeld, 1954; Little, 1958; Searles, 1963; Kernberg, 1984). Schizophrenic patients are more vulnerable still. They have a very difficult time distinguishing between the therapist as a transference figure and as a real object. Little (1958) has called such transferences "delusional." Part of the basis for the changing and inconstant object images of the therapist has to do with the schizophrenic's tendency to fuse self and object representations, and to use primitive forms of projection which blur self and object boundaries (Kernberg, 1975). It is unclear as to who is the patient, who is the therapist, and what belongs to each.

Some writers have suggested that one must not confront the schizophrenic patient with his delusional perceptions, if at all possible (Walder, 1925; Clark, 1933; Balint, 1959; Spotnitz, 1969). Balint (1959) has written that the therapist, "should not be an entity in his own right . . . in fact, not a sharply contoured object at all, but should blend into the friendly expanses surrounding the patient" (p. 97). The aim of this blending in is to form a "narcissistic alliance" with the patient and to gradually "draw the patient out" into the object world.

With schizophrenic patients this strategy is often impossible if not counterproductive. Precisely because of the patient's ego modifications and primitive defenses, he often cannot make use of direct support. His mistrust and envy (Klein, 1957) spoil incoming nourishment; as often as not, the patient sees attempts at support through paranoid lenses: food becomes poison.

Moreover, at least partly because certain psychotic defenses (e.g., fusion of self and object representations, projective identification, psychotic denial) disrupt ego functioning, reality testing breaks down. In order to preserve reality testing, and to reverse the effect of these pathological defenses, it is important that the therapist be very precisely "contoured." Schizophrenic patients often need a sharply and clearly defined object as a model, and as a kind of trellis against which to develop. The therapist's remaining indistinct and shadowy often leads to confusion and frustration. In any event, many schizophrenic patients will simply continue to press the issue of the patient–therapist boundary until it is either clarified constructively, or the treatment breaks down.

Ms. Williams, the young woman from the inner city, was in Dr. C's office and, again, tried to unplug the telephone and answering machine.

Dr. C: In my office, you behave as if my things are your things. As if my office and body belong to you. If I stop you, it upsets you and you begin to feel some kind of pain. But if I don't, I feel pain because you act as if what is mine belongs to you. You want to block out your suffering by being a clown with me. You feel better if you make our relationship into a joke, and block me out.

Ms. W: With my family, I did the same thing.

At this point, Dr. C explained to the patient that they would hold their meetings on the inpatient unit and not in her private office, and that she would ask a staff member to observe them, if Ms. Williams could not refrain from disrupting sessions.

Ms. W: You're saying that John and Robert (members of the staff) will be in session with us?

Dr. C: Yes.

Ms. Williams leaned back, smiled, and then got up to unplug the lamp.

Dr. C: When you act this way, I take it to mean that you want to destroy me, my office, and the treatment. Maybe you wonder why I sit here calmly, while you try to destroy me. Maybe you wonder if I'm crazy or if I want you to hurt me. Well, I don't want you to hurt me, and I'm not crazy. From now on, we'll have to meet on the unit, not in my private office anymore. If I have to, I'll ask the staff to join us so we'll both know that you won't be able to harm me or my things.

In this example, Dr. C set a limit with the patient specifically related to the location of the boundary between them. Dr. C did not allow Ms. Williams to continue to invade her privacy or destroy her property. Dr. C presented the patient with a "sharp contour" in relation to which she could learn more about her therapist and herself. Clearly, Ms. Williams pushed Dr. C to the point where it was impossible for her not to do this. I think that many schizophrenic patients need the therapist to define his identity in certain areas in order to begin to define themselves, and often force the therapist's hand in this direction.

Sometimes, becoming a defined object involves sharing feelings with the patient.

Ms. W: I'm frightened. Sometimes, I think of beating my sister with a rock. Or of shooting my brother. If I pulled a gun on you would you be frightened?

Dr. C: Yes.

Sometimes, realistic acknowledgment of the patient's effect on one's feelings clarifies the boundary between patient and therapist, and can facilitate the patient's expression of feeling. Ms. Williams had talked incoherently for quite awhile, but finally was speaking in a more direct and poignant way about her sadness.

Dr. C: You know, when we talk together, I feel upset. When you tell me your feelings, I feel sad. Even though it hurts sometimes, it's a lot better than when you were out of control and making a joke out of our relationship. Now, when you talk, it makes sense to me. How do you feel about it?

Mr. DeVito had spent months in the treatment acting as if he were formless and without an identity.

Mr. D: You know, when I walked in today, I thought I saw you looking out the window with a sad and forlorn expression. I thought at first that I must be mistaken. That you couldn't be feeling that way.
Dr. B: Why not?
Mr. D: Because you seem like such a together person. It just didn't seem to make sense that you were feeling sad. But I also thought, if he feels that way sometimes, maybe he could see what I'm going through. Was I right? Were you sad?
Dr. B: I think you did pick something up. There have been some unhappy things that have happened to me recently, and I guess it shows up on my face. What you picked up was accurate.

Mr. D: I feel like a human being.

Dr. B: How so?

Mr. D: Like I can talk about feelings like a real person, and that I know what's going on.

Mr. DeVito went on in the session to discuss feelings of emptiness and isolation from others.

Part of the value in selectively expressing one's opinions or feelings to the patient is that it can help him to evaluate the accuracy of his testing of reality. In this case, Mr. DeVito did correctly identify the mood that led to his therapist's sad expression. To acknowledge this to Mr. DeVito, whose reality testing was often impaired, not only did no harm, but helped him to develop confidence in his capacity to observe and understand others. Not to have acknowledged the correctness of his perception would have been to have lost a chance to confirm his capacity for empathy.

Emotional Induction

Awareness. Scores of psychoanalytic writers have discussed the nonverbal process by which the therapist's emotions resonate with the subjective emotional experience of the patient, even though these feelings may not be in the patient's awareness. Such therapist reactions may yield insight into the patient's mental life which can be gained in no other way (Rosenfeld, 1952; Semrad, Manaer, Mann, and Standish, 1952; Beres and Arlow, 1974). Little (1957, 1958) has specified populations of patients in which this occurs particularly often: psychotic patients, patients with certain character disorders, patients with psychosomatic conditions, and patients who have difficulty putting thoughts and feelings into words.

My impression is that there is an inverse relation between the patient's capacity to identify and communicate inner emotional states and his use of nonverbal methods to convey his feelings. I have referred to this nonverbal form of communication as "emotional induction" (Lotterman, 1990). It is as if the less the patient is able to use words as vehicles to transmit meanings, the more he relies upon this nonverbal inducing of emotions to communicate with the therapist. In psychoanalytic therapy with neurotics, the therapist's use of his own emotional reactions to guide his understanding of the patient can complement his cognitive insight. In work with schizophrenic patients, these therapist reactions are indispensable and may be the only way the patient's inner life can enter the treatment at all. Such patients may talk little or do so in largely incoherent or disconnected ways, leaving the therapist few verbal clues as to what is going on. However, a patient often will act in a way that puts the therapist in an emotional position similar to his own.

In work with neurotics, one feels one's attention directed to ideas and feelings which, phenomenologically, feel "over there," somehow psychologically localized near the patient. Whether it is an emotion, a fantasy, or a thought, it is as if one is a member of an audience watching the action on a separate stage. One has the psychic room to reflect, to muse, to allow one's mind to wander. One feels emotionally responsive, but not immediately involved in the action. In other words, there is some emotional distance.

In work with borderline patients, and especially schizophrenic patients, the "location" of the action of the treatment often feels very different. One frequently feels that psychological phenomena, often intense and disturbing, are "over here," inside oneself, while the patient remains calm, unperturbed, and unreflective. It feels as if one is no longer watching a drama at leisure. Rather, one feels that the actors have come down off the stage and have drawn one into the performance. As might happen in the theater, if, for example, a comic draws one into the act, one feels as if the action is going on, not "over there," but "over here," all around and inside oneself. It is by translating this intense emotional experience into words and concepts that the therapist may come to understand more about the transference.

Ms. Williams, whose antics disrupted her sessions with Dr. C and led Dr. C to bring staff members into their meetings, had been trying, once again, to put on Dr. C's coat and unplug her answering machine. One day, Dr. C was feeling particularly intruded upon and helpless. She felt that her privacy had been invaded and that everything was topsy-turvy. As she was just coming to recognize these feelings during a session with Ms. Williams, the patient said: "You're trying to drive me insane. You want to make me all confused." Apparently, with her unpredictable antics, Ms. Williams managed to induce very similar feelings in Dr. C about her.

On another occasion, Ms. Williams had kept Dr. C waiting at a time when they urgently needed to talk.

Dr. C: I feel frustrated. I was eager to start our session, but I felt I didn't have any control over when you'd get here.

Ms. W: Control is something I *never* have here. Patients on this unit never have a say over anything. *Now you feel some of what I go through everyday.*

Mr. DeVito, the man beset with the gangster, had few thoughts, feelings, or wishes for months. His therapist and he had spent many sessions together with seemingly very little of value going on. The therapist felt torpid, useless, and that his identity as a professional had dissolved. He felt uncomfortably formless and passive. Since this had become such a powerful part of his experience with Mr. DeVito, and since he had few other clinical clues to help him understand what was going on, the therapist shared this reaction with the patient.

Dr. B: I want to let you know what I'm feeling. My feelings may tell us something about what's going on in you. Sometimes when we meet I feel very tired and slow, like my mind is in a fog. I feel like my mind has shut down, that my thoughts and feelings are empty and sometimes I can't remember what I'm supposed to be doing here. At times, I feel like sitting back and daydreaming, hoping that nothing interrupts it. It feels cozy and blank.

Mr. D: I feel like that all the time.

Mr. DeVito went on to talk about how he felt like a "lump" and had no clear sense of his own identity or value. He expressed anger at the therapist for describing how he felt, and for giving up on him. He understood the purpose of Dr. B's remarks, however, and over the next several weeks was able to explore his feelings of worthlessness, passivity, and emptiness. Considerable behavioral change also followed.

Later, I will discuss in more detail the value and timing of sharing induced emotions with the patient, but here, I would like to emphasize how Mr. DeVito had managed to convey a very complicated experience to the therapist without the use of words. Moreover, the therapist's grasp of Mr. DeVito's emotional situation was not an abstract one. He had an immediate experience of what worthlessness, formlessness, and emptiness meant for the patient.

Mechanism. Despite the recent focus on the way in which the patient's emotions are communicated via the "total" countertransference (Kernberg, 1975, 1984), many authors remain puzzled about how this actually occurs. Fenichel (1945) wrote, "We know nothing about the specific nature of this identification" (p. 84). Sullivan (1953) wrote, "The rationale of this induction—that is, how anxiety in the mothering one, induces anxiety in the infant—is thoroughly obscure." Kernberg (1984) noted, "We probably still do not know enough about how one person's behavior may induce emotional and behavioral reactions in another" (p. 123).

A number of writers have turned to the concept of "projective identification" as an explanation for the way in which the patient's feelings appear to be induced in the therapist. There are several problems with this explanation. First, the term *projective identification* is used so variously that few agree on a precise meaning. Originally (Klein, 1946), it referred to an *intrapsychic fantasy* in which bad parts of the self were split off and forced into another person. The term did not have an interpersonal aspect until Bion (1956) described the way in which the patient would so treat the therapist that the latter became a "container" for the patient's fantasy, and somehow came to experience some of the fantasied contents himself. Still later, the term was used rather promiscuously, and came at different times to refer to a fantasy, a defense, an object relation, a mode of communication, and a pathway for change (Ogden, 1979). Kulish (1985) wrote of the term's ambiguity and overinclusiveness: "To ask a concept to be a fantasy, a defense, and an object relationship, is to ask it to do too much" (p. 91). Because projective identification has lost much of its conceptual clarity, its value as an explanation has been undermined.

The second problem with explaining induced emotion by

means of projective identification is that no explanation has really been advanced. The term is invoked, but no one has accounted for how it works. That is to say, no mechanism has been described. What does one person actually do to another to evoke particular feelings and fantasies? How is emotional experience transmitted between two people without the use of words? How can such communication occur unconsciously?

I would like to propose the following explanation, which I presented in much greater detail in an earlier paper (Lotterman, 1990). Both Bion (1959) and Searles (1979) have described the way in which patients can purposefully, even if unconsciously, play upon the therapist's feelings. In particular, Searles noted that some of his patients felt that their parents had tried to communicate their own internal states by putting them in certain similar, real interpersonal situations. These patients believed that their parents were intentionally communicating to them in this way.

I believe that a mechanism such as this occurs frequently in psychotherapy. Patients behave in characteristic ways which are designed to generate predictable emotional reactions in the therapist. The process is similar to that used by actors when they wish to produce predictable dramatic effects in their audiences. Hamlet berated Guildenstern for playing upon him in just such a way.

> You would play upon me, you would seem to know my stops, you would pluck out the heart of my mystery, you would sound me from my lowest note to the top of my compass; and there is much music, excellent voice, in this little organ, yet cannot you make it speak. 'Sblood, do you think I am easier to be played on than a pipe? (Act III, Scene ii).

Skillful playwrights know that intellectual speeches do not generate intense emotions in the audience. They *arrange* sequences of actions, words, and expressions in order to generate expectable emotional responses. T. S. Eliot wrote in "Hamlet and His Problems" (1919), "The only way of expressing emotion in the form of art is by finding an 'objective correlative'; in other words a *set of objects, a situation, a chain of events* which shall be the formula for that *particular* emotion" (quoted in Bartlett [1980], p. 809; emphasis added).

When Ms. Williams said, "Now you feel what I feel" I think she was acknowledging the fact that she had put her therapist in an emotional position similar to her own, and that as a result Dr. C had come to feel what it was like to be her. In the examples described above, the patients used techniques and tools similar to those used in the theater: *mime, stage management* (the sequencing and location of action), *delivery* (consisting of *timing* and *tone*) *costume*, and *props*. All these nonverbal techniques helped to provoke, arouse, and stimulate feelings and thereby add force to the emotional position the patient was trying to impress on the therapist.

One might say that such *induced emotion* is the executive arm of projective identification defined strictly as a fantasy. When induced emotion occurs together with fantasies of entry and control (Klein, 1946), it can mold the external environment in the image of the internal, so that the individual's interpersonal world has been altered to resemble his fantasies. (A more detailed explanation of the mechanism of induced emotions is given earlier [Lotterman, 1990].)

Disclosure. How does one make therapeutic use of emotions induced by the patient? Some authors advise against disclosing feelings to the patient under all circumstances (Heimann, 1950), and simply suggest that the therapist use this countertransference information as part of his general store of knowledge about the patient. I believe that disclosing one's emotional response can be very useful with schizophrenic patients, if one's personal reactions and responses are carefully monitored. As I have discussed in the sections on parameters and object definition, sharing one's reactions with the patient is often an essential aspect of setting needed limits. Beyond this, however, a patient may act in such a way toward the therapist as to induce reactions which can seem improper or unseemly to discuss with the patient. The therapist may feel disgusted by the patient, revolted or contemptuous. He may feel sadistic or enraged or loving or longing. Much psychotherapy training teaches us not to communicate such feelings for fear of burdening or confusing the patient.

In work with schizophrenic patients, however, the therapist's reaction is often the first, if not the only way for essential transference material to enter the treatment. The example of Dr. B's discussion with Mr. DeVito was such a case. It is as if the therapist were the patient's auxiliary ego, with the following distinct functions: affect tolerance, affect recognition, concept formation, symbol (word) selection, and communication. The therapist, in locum tenens so to speak, thus becomes the integrator, concept former, and communicator of the feelings that the patient has induced in him. To *not* communicate these emotions, at times, is to be drawn into the patient's resistance to these affects. A sophisticated, even if seemingly disorganized patient may use his therapist's professional reticence to act outrageously toward him, and this may serve as a haven for resistance (Freud, 1916–1917). Such emotions either become lost or are so attenuated by euphemistic references to them, that they have no mutative therapeutic effect. Patients often rely on their own denial of internal and external reality, primitive projection, and desymbolization (Searles, 1965) to keep ideas and feelings from registering emotionally. Patients may also use the therapist's verbal restraint, based on a desire to remain "neutral," "abstinent," or "tactful," as an ally to exclude ideas and feelings which need to be discussed openly and understood. The patient's exposure to a reasonably well-integrated ego such as the therapist's, can help him discover in what way he is similar to others and different from them. It can help him distinguish between what is inside and what is outside, what is self and what is other (Kernberg, 1975). Thus it can be a powerful catalyst for the growth of the capacity to test reality.

The therapist's disclosure of his own reactions is often very important in establishing a positive interpersonal relationship—the "pact" that Freud spoke of. For patients who have little experience in connecting feelings to thoughts, and thoughts to behavior, and who use various disintegrative mechanisms to fend off the emotional meanings that occur when such connections are made, it is important to encounter another person who makes such meaningful links. This does not mean that the therapist must disclose material about his personal past, although at times, as in the example of Mr. DeVito, this may be helpful, if the therapist is comfortable doing so. It does often mean that the therapist may say what is on his mind, especially as it relates to the treatment setting.

In addition, it is important to keep in mind that one's emotional response to the patient is not always generated by one's own, unique emotional makeup. The behavior of some patients would stir up a similar emotional response, for example, anger, in any "average expectable" observer. Winnicott coined the term *objective countertransference* for such expectable reactions to the patient. If this is so in any particular case, it is very important that the patient understand his impact on the feelings and attitudes of others. Disclosing induced emotion can help in this process.

Several objections might be made to sharing one's emotions with the patient, especially if he is psychotic. Won't the patient feel burdened by hearing about the therapist's inner life? Won't the patient take these emotional expressions literally and feel that he is the "real" object of the therapist who hates or loves him? Won't the patient feel that the therapist has forsaken his "objective" therapeutic role? In work with psychotic patients, won't disclosing induced emotions that seem magically to cross over from one person to another, serve to erode the boundary between therapist and patient, a boundary which above all, should be clear and distinct? While all these concerns are legitimate and understandable in theory, they are not born out in practice.

Occasionally, a patient may have a strong reaction to the therapist's sharing of his feelings. When I told one patient that I felt "overwhelmed," she worried that she had burdened me. Another woman felt that she had hurt me, or that my telling her that I felt "confused" meant that I wanted to get rid of her. When I explained that the reason why I was telling her about my own feelings was because these reactions might be signals telling us about her emotional state, the patient was well able to understand and work productively. It is often useful to explain the purpose of disclosure to the patient in advance.

Should the therapist be completely "candid" and "honest" about all his reactions? If he feels contempt, disgust, fear, or sexual arousal, should he share these reactions with the patient? If so much emotional information enters the treatment via the countertransference, and if attention to the interpersonal relationship is so vital, can one afford *not* to share these feelings with the patient?

As a practical matter, I think, the answer to this last question is yes. To begin with, when emotions first come into the therapist's awareness it is not clear what they signify. Annoyance or disgust, for example, may be defensive against growing affection for the patient. The therapist's reactions must be understood before they can be disclosed in a therapeutically useful way. Also, a particular countertransference affect or thought and its transference implications, may not be the most salient material at that point. At times, the therapist's responses, even painful ones, may be essential to introduce, but the ultimate criterion for doing so is whether this will be therapeutically useful.

Moreover, the therapist is not free of the obligation to consider whether his "induced emotions" actually reflect emotional reactions based on his own past, and not the patient's. I think that with a reasonable degree of self-awareness, though, the therapist can distinguish between what belongs to him, and what to the patient.

Ms. Jackson was the schizophrenic woman in her early twenties who lived with her aunt and uncle, the Tafts. She had extremely poor impulse control and spent hours hanging around the town park. After a great deal of discussion and painstaking negotiation, her therapist and she agreed that she would take medication for her psychotic symptoms. She reported for over two weeks that she had faithfully followed the treatment plan. Her therapist then learned from her family that Ms. Jackson had lied about taking her medication, and in fact, had taken none. This development had been preceded by an episode in which the patient had taken a journal from the therapist's hallway closet.

Dr. S: I want to talk with you about your not taking the medication we agreed on. It makes me very angry.

Ms. J: I know, I know. (as if to brush it aside)

Dr. S: What I'm going to say you may be able to guess already, but I think it's good for me to say it directly to you. Being silent about this, and keeping my feelings in, are not going to help. I don't want to put you down or attack you, but I do want to let you know what I'm feeling. When you took my journal from me, I felt you were saying that you didn't respect me or my feelings. I do my best to respect you and what you're telling me, but I felt like you were saying that my feelings don't matter to you and it made me angry. In this situation, when I found out that you weren't taking the medicine, but were telling me that you were, it seemed you didn't care if you told me the truth or not. I said to myself, "I'm trying to be honest with her, and to help her as best as I can, but she thinks so little of me, she doesn't even bother to tell me the truth." Do you see why I felt this way?

Although the patient initially did not want to discuss her stealing and lying, the therapist's disclosing her feelings did bring them into focus. The patient and therapist were able to go on to discuss the patient's anger, devaluation, and her sense of helplessness that anything, whether it was medication, job training, or psychotherapy could help her feel better.

Over a number of months, Ms. Williams had begun to participate well in her psychotherapy. Her former provocative antics had subsided, but Dr. C had recently told her that she would be graduating from her training program, and, so, would leave the unit for another position in the hospital. In the wake of that announcement, the patient missed several sessions. When Dr. C and she met, Dr. C asked her about the connection between her absence and her feelings. Dr. C commented that perhaps Ms. Williams had missed the sessions because it would stir up painful feelings about Dr. C's leaving the unit. She shrugged off both Dr. C's comments and remained mocking and uninterested.

Dr. C: I want to tell you something. I actually felt relieved when we didn't meet. Thinking it over, why might I have felt relieved?

Ms. W: Maybe you were busy. Maybe they wanted you over in the nurse's station. Maybe you didn't want to see me.

Dr. C: Well, the real reason is because talking about stopping our sessions makes me feel sad. It is painful to think about. And sometimes, I guess a part of me would rather not think about it, or feel it, so that I don't have to feel so upset. But that's only one side of me. The rest wanted to meet with you and talk about what is going on between us. That part of me was unhappy that we didn't meet.

Ms. W: When you go I'll feel alone and sad. They'll want to give me a new therapist. But it won't be the same. I don't want someone new. I just want to work with you.

Ms. Williams began the session with a flippant nonchalance. She was not willing to put her emotions into words, and did not respond to the therapist's cognitive linking of the missed session and her being upset. It seemed to Dr. C. that when she described her own emotional reaction, however, which was so similar to the patient's, that it was more difficult for the patient to remain flip and detached.

Sometimes the emotion induced in the therapist reflects the patient's feelings about some important figure in his life. Here is an example from work with a borderline man.

The patient, Richard Martin, had been talking about how unhappy he was in life. He was particularly upset with his girl friend, whom he described as an irresponsible woman who always got herself into jams, and who expected the patient to bail her out. He complained that she never took the responsibility for making changes. Mr. Martin went on to say how he had been telling all his friends how bad his life was, while actually doing very little to help himself.

Mr. M: Everything sucks. I was telling two guys on my softball team, Daryl and Howard, about how everything is falling apart.

Dr. R: What made you tell them about it?

Mr. M: I don't know.

There is a pause, while the therapist thinks about this.

Mr. M: It's almost like I'm waiting for you to say something to make it all better. I feel like a little bird with its mouth open for food.

Dr. R: What's that like?

Mr. M: It makes me feel fragile, and lost.

Dr. R: You know, I'm feeling as if I have to do all the work. And also annoyed. It feels like all these things are happening to you and that you're not willing to make an effort for yourself.

Mr. Martin thinks for awhile.

Mr. M: I feel just the same way with Caroline, my girl friend.

Dr. R: You keep on rescuing her every time she gets herself in a jam. How come?

Mr. M: I don't know. Maybe I feel powerful if I can make someone else feel guilty or responsible for me and then get them to take care of my problems. Maybe I feel that if I'm in pain, I have the right to demand that people bail me out. And that's better than solving my own problems. I guess that somehow, I let Caroline do this kind of thing to me.

When the therapist discusses his own emotions, especially painful or powerful ones, this can help the patient to understand that feelings are not necessarily as dangerous or overwhelming as they may first seem. Most schizophrenic patients are frightened of their affects. For a patient to hear the therapist discuss his own feelings can demonstrate that it is possible to feel, contain, and verbalize emotion. In this regard, the therapist's disclosure serves as a model.

Ms. W: Sometimes when we meet I feel uptight, nervous.

Dr. C: Sometimes I feel uptight and nervous too.

Ms. W: How come?

Dr. C: Because sometimes I don't know what's going to happen between us. How you're going to act, or whether you'll make a joke out of everything, or even if you're going to come.

Ms. W: Well, I guess everybody is nervous some of the time.

Ms. Williams, again, was angry at her therapist for leaving the unit. She said that she was afraid to talk about her feelings. Dr. C and she talked for awhile about her fear. Then Dr. C commented:

Dr. C: You know, I had the same reaction when we began working together. When you were reaching for my clothes, and unplugging the lamp and the answering machine, I felt angry but I kept it in because I thought that afterwards, you wouldn't want to speak with me. I was nervous about that. After awhile, I began to think more clearly. But it wasn't easy for me.

Ms. W: To tell you the truth, I feel like you're walking out on me. Like everyone does.

Sharing emotional reactions with the patient does not necessarily involve painful or unpleasant feelings.

Deborah Weiss, whose apathy, lack of energy, and poverty of affect were almost unbudgable, brought a book of quotations to her session. She read a very poignant quote from Robert Frost on the need for love. Her reading sent chills through Dr. E, her therapist. Dr. E's eyes filled with tears. Dr. E told the patient about his reaction, and this led to a discussion of how emotionally dead the patient felt, and of her fears of feeling. In the sessions that followed, she was more expressive and responsive.

Naming

Since all verbal psychotherapy rests on the patient's capacity to use words, the disturbance of symbol use is a particularly debilitating problem. When thought is incoherent and language use fragmented, there are no vehicles to carry emotional meaning between the patient and the therapist. Two related techniques are designed to address this problem. Over a period of time they seem to promote change in the thought and language disturbance of psychotic patients.

Many of these patients have trouble putting their thoughts and feelings into words (Little, 1958). When asked how they feel, many patients say that their minds are blank. Some answer with concrete or somatic imagery: "I'm tired"; "I have a headache"; "My body is changed." Some produce a solitary word such as *awful* underneath which sits a continent of affect and thought. Ms. Weiss said that her emotions were "too submerged, too far underground" to utter. Ms. Bender said that it was "tough to get a hold of an idea and bring it to my lips." (In chapter 6, I will suggest some ideas about why there is a disconnection between verbal symbols and affect.)

The technique of naming consists of a systematic, meticulous, and, at times, seemingly labored focus on the patient's choice and use of words. The patient may allude to an affect indirectly. Or, it may seem to the therapist that an affect would fit in a certain context, but is absent from the patient's account. The therapist may ask the patient how he feels, and is not deterred by the patient's "I don't know" or "I can't think." The patient may be at a loss for affective terms for his inner states and, at the outset, may only offer descriptions of physical sensations. That is a start. Instead of loneliness or loss, the patient may feel queasy, or have a lump in his throat. Instead of feeling humiliated and that his self-image has been injured, he may feel that his appearance has been changed. In place of feeling manipulated by the therapist, he may have the sensation of something tugging at his neck.

Each description, if it is noted, and if the patient is encouraged to expand upon it, can lead to further associative links. At first, these may remain concrete and somatic. Nevertheless, this can be productive as long as the patient begins to learn and practice the process of connecting words (no matter how poor their initial accuracy) with internal states. Often, a patient who begins by describing a physical sensation can eventually identify underlying emotions.

Ms. Williams had just returned from the funeral of a relative. She cared for this woman, and Dr. C assumed that she would feel sad.

Ms. W: We went to the funeral. I saw her and felt a heavy feeling in my heart.
Dr. C: If you were a movie director, and I was an actor, and you were trying to help me feel what you feel, what would you say?
Ms. W: I'd say you'd have to have tears in your eyes, and you'd have to cry and feel very sorrowful.

On another occasion, Ms. Williams returned to the hospital after a visit with friends. She said that she was homesick for her friends and did not want to come back to the hospital. At this point, Ms. Williams could rarely identify or express her feelings. Since she alluded to an emotion (i.e., "homesick"), Dr. C decided to follow up.

Ms. W: I felt like I was cooped up here in the hospital. Like
           there is nothing for me here. It's empty here. Every-
           thing for me is back home.

Dr. C: You mentioned feeling homesick. Tell me as much as
           you can about what it's like to feel homesick. If you were
           a poet, and put it in the words with the most feeling in
           them, what would you say?

Ms. W: I'd say that it's like a wound. It makes me suffer. Like
           I'm stranded and there's no one around. It's not an
           actual wound; it's worse than that. It's a wound to my
           feelings.

Roger DeVito began a session by discussing how he had sat by himself at work in the employees' lounge. Dr. B asked the patient to help him understand what it was like to be in his shoes, by painting a picture of his experience in words. Mr. DeVito began by describing a warm, unpleasant sensation in his chest, "heartburn" as he called it. As he and his therapist focused more and more on the details of these physical sensations, and as he became more and more precise about them, affect-laden words slowly began to emerge, and he was able to realize how irritated he felt at his boss. He said he often felt "hot under the collar," and said that he was afraid that his angry feelings might explode.

Mr. DeVito began a session by saying that he felt out of touch with Dr. B.

Mr. D: I feel hollow inside. Like there is nothing. Also, it is as
           if there is nothing coming in from the outside. It's as
           if there is a shield around me.

Dr. B: Describe the shield in as much detail as you can.

Mr. D: It's as if it's a beautiful spring day, and it's cool but the
           sun is shining and making everything warm. But I can't
           get warm. Something blocks the sun.

Dr. B: You'd like to feel the warmth.

Mr. D: The warm feeling doesn't get through.

Dr. B: So, the shield mainly blocks sensations coming from
           outside you. It's not mainly a shield against what you
           feel inside.

Mr. D: Right. The sunshine doesn't touch me. You know, I
           don't feel I have contact with anyone, maybe I have a

kind of feeling against letting them in. Maybe it's a
shield against people.

Dr. B: You would like to have some warm contact, like feeling
the sunshine on your skin, but it also frightens you. You
have told me how you feel so easily hurt by your friends,
and how much pain you have felt. Maybe this shield is
to protect you against that kind of pain.

Mr. D: And also my aunt and uncle. They don't know how to
comfort me. They're always so rough and hard.

Dr. B: You'd like some contact with people to feel warmer,
but you're afraid it will hurt you instead, and so you
need a shield.

Mr. D: Right.

This last example illustrates several important ideas. First,
one must take the notion of psychic determinism seriously
enough to want to pursue Mr. DeVito's allusion to a shield. One
must assume that Mr. DeVito's word choice at that moment was
not capricious or meaningless—that possibly it functioned as a
"switch" word (Freud, 1905) representing a link between several
trains of unconscious thought. These are expressions which strike
the listener's ear as being out of place, unique, or singular in
some way. Freud believed that they represent "nodal points"
(Breuer and Freud, 1895, p. 290) at which two or more streams
of unconscious thought converge. These points are often marked
by notable or singular verbal usages. One must assume that each
additional image (e.g., sunshine, getting warm) carries specific
meaning. For example, it may be significant that Mr. DeVito described the shield as being one against an external stimulus. This
attention to the details of the patient's speech may seem pedantic
and overdone and can sometimes feel tedious when put into practice. Nevertheless, it can bear a great deal of fruit, especially with
patients who say they have no thoughts or feelings at all and who
appear devoid of an internal life.

Enlargement

The technique of enlargement is linked to that of naming, and,
in a sense, is an extension of it, but it assumes a broader lexicon
of affective language. Once a patient has at least some capacity

to attach words to subjective ideas and feelings, enlargement can be used to explore the patient's associations. I use the term *enlargement* to make a rough analogy to the process of magnifying photographs—the details of the image are expanded so that it can be seen more clearly. This technique, like clarification, involves asking the patient to "say more." Unlike free association, it focuses the patient on the task of verbal description in a more methodical way. If the patient feels like breaking off a description or association, sometimes (although not always) he is encouraged to pursue it anyway. If the patient has no more ideas on a subject, he may be asked nevertheless to continue to put his thoughts into words. This technique might be called "focused" or "directed" association. The purpose of enlargement is to reverse the process of breaking links (Bion, 1959) between important and related groups of ideas and feelings. The associations of psychotic patients are often broken down, or blocked; one idea does not evoke another. This breakdown of meaningful links is more marked than in neurosis. Amongst these patients idea and emotion are barren and fruitless; they stop dead in their associative tracks. If a schizophrenic patient who begins by saying that his mind is empty or that he has "no thoughts" is encouraged to expand on the sensations and images he does have, sometimes a good deal of affect and fantasy will emerge.

Ms. Thompson was a psychotic woman in her midtwenties who generally was unable to verbalize her feelings, and left the impression that her inner life was quite impoverished and empty. On this day, she seemed filled with unspoken emotion.

Ms. T: I wish I was far away with no worries. No hassles.

Dr. D: Tell me in as much detail as you can about what you wish. I'm very interested. Let's imagine that I was a magician and granted you all your wishes. What would they be? Take as much time as you like, and don't leave anything out.

Ms. T: Well, first I'd be the queen of a medieval kingdom, and I'd have a huge castle with spiral staircase. I'd be the absolute authority, and I'd have lots of servants.

Dr. D: How many?

Ms. T: A hundred. No, two hundred. And everyone would curry favor with me. If I was displeased, I'd send them to the dungeon.

Dr. D: Your subjects, how would they feel about you? Would
           you want them to be afraid, or adore you for being
           kind, or what?

Ms. T: I'd be the one who gave out the food. So everyone
           would obey me and respect me. If someone disobeyed,
           I'd send them to the dungeon without food, and where
           everything was silent. There would be no sounds, no
           music, and the guards wouldn't be allowed to speak
           with them.

Dr. D: They would be alone, cut off from people?

Ms. T: Completely.

Dr. D: Cutting them off from people would make them suffer.

Ms. T: A lot. Then they'd lose all their feelings. They wouldn't
           be able to feel anything anymore.

Dr. D: So, let's go over what you've told me up to this point.
           As queen, you'd rule a kingdom and live in a huge
           castle. You would be in control, and if your subjects
           disobeyed, you'd punish them by sending them to a
           dungeon where there would be no sound, and no peo-
           ple. That would make them suffer. Finally, they'd lose
           their feelings.

Ms. T: Exactly.

Dr. D: If you were cut off like that from people how would it
           make you feel?

Ms. T: It would be bleak. Like being insane. There would be
           no one and nothing. I couldn't stand it. I'd try to tune
           everything out.

In the discussion that followed, Ms. Thompson began to talk
about her own sense of isolation and her perception that her
therapist was withholding and controlling. The therapist chose
the subject of isolation and the deadening of feelings for expan-
sion because these experiences were important and painful for
the patient.

Enlargement is similar in some ways to Freud's early pressure
technique in which he actively encouraged patients to associate
to certain symptoms or events (Breuer and Freud, 1985, pp.
270–280). The pressure technique with its emphasis on hypnosis,
gave way to a more open-ended form of association which Freud
called "free association." For neurotic patients, whose cognitive

links, conscious and unconscious, are reasonably intact, the main impediment to full conscious recall is resistance based on the repression of such links. In schizophrenic patients, it seems that further violence has been done to associative bonds in the mental apparatus, resulting in blocking, thought stoppage, and looseness of association. It appears that these interruptions in linkage are different in kind from those in neurosis. Unlike neurosis, where only the quality of consciousness is deleted, in schizophrenia, concreteness and disturbances in symbolizing impede verbal and other conceptual forms of cognitive linking. Whatever the mechanism, with schizophrenic patients a structured effort at associating can be helpful.

This technique rests on recognizing emotionally charged words and phrases. Roger DeVito[1] had been feeling frustrated and painfully agitated.

Mr. D: I have bad heartburn.

Dr. B: How do you mean? Do you feel that your heart is burning?

Mr. D: I mean that everything is moving inside. Like it's roasting. It's like nothing soothes me. I feel like my heart is roasting, that it's hot and I can't cool it down. I'm irritable with myself, with you and with everybody. So I stay away from people.

Dr. B: So that your anger doesn't get too hot?

Mr. D: Yeah. I guess my anger is pretty intense sometimes.

Deborah Weiss said that her feelings had been "interred." This struck Dr. E as a curious way for her to express herself. When Dr. E asked her what "interred" meant, she had a hard time explaining. She said that it was just an expression. Dr. E asked her if she meant "interred" in the sense of dead, as one would inter a body that was no longer alive. Or, did she mean "interred" in the sense that something might be located under a great deal of material, but that it still existed, and was perhaps still alive. Or was she using the word *interred* to refer to being trapped beneath a great obstacle which had to be removed for her to be free of

---

[1]Mr. DeVito had an extensive neurological workup for unrelated reasons. This workup included a CAT scan and an EEG. The results were negative.

it? As Ms. Weiss and Dr. E explored these various possibilities about what the patient initially claimed was "just an expression," information emerged about how she felt cut off from people, how her feelings no longer seemed alive, and how helpless and hopeless she felt about ever being "discovered" (or "disinterred") by anyone after so many years trapped in her emotional isolation. *Interred* actually turned out to be quite an apt term to summarize her experience.

Enlargement is a technique designed to help the patient express otherwise nonintegrated thoughts and feelings. It is an extension of the usual technique of clarification used in psychoanalytic therapy. Obviously, it should not be used in such a way as to seem inquisitorial or persecutory (Olinick, 1954). Too frequent questions can sometimes make a patient feel put on the spot. This technique should be used tactfully in the context of a collaborative effort.

The use of enlargement or directed association will appear to be worth the labor of picking up associative threads with sometimes recalcitrant or distracted patients, only if one takes the concept of psychic determinism seriously. All the words the patient uses, and each expression, must be taken as potentially vital signs on a treasure map, marking where to dig further. The example involving Ms. Bender's hallucination of the rasping sound given at the beginning of the chapter is, I think, a good one. The seeming disintegration of the patient's intentional speech should not deter us from being alert to nodal points. Patience and tenacity are very often rewarded.

Building the Therapeutic Relationship

The Negative Interpersonal Reaction. As I mentioned at the outset of this chapter, whether the interpersonal relationship and the transference are different or the same is a matter of debate (Brenner, 1980). For this discussion, I will treat the interpersonal relationship and the transference as separate but related phenomena. The term *interpersonal relationship* will refer to vicissitudes of the current interaction between patient and therapist, albeit colored by transference and countertransference. One of the implications of discriminating between these two concepts is that some element in the therapist–patient dyad may be experienced as "new," "unique," or "real" to the patient, distinct from his past experience or transference expectations. This may, for example, include a correct perception about the therapist's emotional state. In any event, the schizophrenic patient often responds to events in a concrete way. Even if a feeling or perception originates from a transference reaction, it often must be dealt with as a real and concrete experience first. We hope that it can be connected to its past origins at some point. Thus, it is often unavoidable that the patient's emotional reactions be treated as if they are current interpersonal experiences. When they are examined, the distortions which emerge may lead to an exploration of what may be underlying the experience.

Perhaps the most important technical requirement in work with schizophrenics is to be in touch with changes in the interpersonal relationship. This relationship can be the first and final obstacle to the psychotherapy process, or it can be the tie, built up by human contact and shared effort, which can lift the work up into something that more and more approaches traditional verbal psychotherapy. The direction the treatment takes often depends on how the interpersonal relationship is monitored and what the therapist does at important moments.

For Freud, one of the sticking points in the psychotherapy of schizophrenia was that the patient could not observe a therapeutic "pact," in today's language, a "therapeutic alliance" (Freud, 1940, p. 173). The patient was too unpredictable and his powers of observation too erratic. His willingness to obey the rules of treatment based on his expectation of love from the analyst was too ephemeral. I do not agree that such a pact is impossible with psychotic patients. But certainly, the alliance with the patient is central to therapeutic success.

As in therapeutic work with other patients, the alliance can be preserved and developed by looking at those things which interfere with its growth. Negative transferences, or, to be consistent, *negative interpersonal reactions*, should be identified, clarified, and either interpreted, explained, or both. If the patient feels kintimidated, overly envious, contemptuous, or ashamed, little work will get done. Attention to these negative interpersonal reactions is essential, and is the first order of business. The therapist should always be asking himself if the patient is feeling spiteful, envious, hopeless, humiliated, or sadistic, and, if so, what he, the therapist, may have done or not done to prompt this response. The patient's willingness to put thoughts and feelings into words will depend on the state of his relationship with the therapist.

The importance of clarifying, confronting, and interpreting the negative transference is also vital. As noted, however, given the often delusional concreteness of the patient, it may be extremely difficult to operate as if this were exclusively a transference matter. The patient's reality testing is not well enough established to appreciate that "everything is transference" (this often is not so easy for healthier patients). Therefore, it is often best to acknowledge what reality there may be behind the patient's reaction if there is one, and then explore what distortions may have been superimposed. If, after exploring both the patient's and the therapist's point of view about what "really happened," the patient can allow the possibility of a distortion, then an attempt to identify a transference reaction can be made.

Mary Williams was looking unhappy. She spoke as if defeated.

Ms. W: Sometimes, *I* feel like sessions make no sense.

Because of the way she emphasized the word, *I*, Dr. C thought that the patient might feel that she, Dr. C, saw things differently.

Dr. C: How do you think *I* feel about the sessions?
Ms. W: *You* seem so clear all the time. You say things that always seem clear and like they make perfect sense. *You* probably think things are going great. That's not what I feel. My thoughts are all jumbled. I don't know what I think or feel half the time.
Dr. C: So, when you're feeling jumbled and confused, I'm acting as if things are clear and simple. How does that make you feel toward me?
Ms. W: Like you don't know anything about what I'm feeling.
Dr. C: What you're saying makes sense to me. Actually, in the last few weeks I've often felt confused and nervous, like I don't know what's going to happen next. For some reason, I felt I shouldn't tell you about that. I don't know why.
Ms. W: That's the way *I* feel all the time.

Dr. C: I'm going to try to understand why I thought I
          shouldn't let myself feel those feelings or talk about
          them with you. I think this is something that would be
          good for us both to work on together.

In the example above, the therapist asked about the patient's
perception of how the therapist regarded the treatment in order
to see why the patient was so listless. She acknowledged the patient's view of her behavior, and explored some of her own emotions and reactions, though not her personal past, unrelated to
the treatment. In doing this, she used disclosure of what was probably an induced emotion, acted like a "contoured" or "defined"
object, and explicitly emphasized the importance of working together with the patient. She thus modeled several attitudes and
behaviors essential for collaborative work.
    As noted, Ms. Williams missed several sessions after Dr. C
told her she would be graduating soon, and leaving the unit to
work elsewhere in the hospital. When she did come, she reverted
to the childish actions and provocative behavior that had first
disrupted her work with Dr. C. Dr. C had expressed her anger to
the patient about this. Ms. Williams had recently become more
serious and able to discuss her sadness.

Dr. C: You know, it's painful to me sometimes when we meet.
          I often feel sad, and it's hard to feel some of these
          feelings. Somehow, I think, you're teaching me to feel
          some of the feelings you have. (The phenomenon of
          emotional induction had been discussed with the pa-
          tient before.) Sometimes it's very painful. But, still, I
          think it's much better than before when you disrupted
          everything. Then, I couldn't think straight and I also
          didn't have a chance to know what I felt. Now, it's more
          serious. My feelings make more sense to me, and I get
          to know what you're feeling better too. I feel more con-
          nected to you.

Supporting the Nonpsychotic Part of the Personality. Many writers
have discussed the significance of the nonpsychotic part of the
personality in working with schizophrenics (Federn, 1934; Katan,
1954; Bion, 1957). This is the only part of the patient that can

form a stable partnership with the therapist in an effort to put feelings into words rather than actions. It is often helpful to refer to this partnership explicitly, to acknowledge the schizophrenic patient's achievements in ways small and large, in engaging in this alliance. This collaborative work is the only ground upon which any ego structure can stand, and its importance cannot be overstated. As Freud (1940) believed, if such a pact cannot be observed no psychotherapy is possible.

Ms. Thompson complained that Dr. D used "ritzy words," and that she didn't understand her. Dr. D appreciated this remark as an effort to make their relationship stronger. Dr. D also felt it was a risk for the patient to admit that she didn't understand her therapist's use of "ritzy words" because of her fear that she was not smart enough.

Ms. T: You use ritzy words. I feel ashamed and dumb because I don't know what you mean.

Dr. D: You're saying that I make you feel even worse about yourself.

Ms. T: Right.

Dr. D: It's very good that you said that. If you can I'd like you to help me stop doing that, and talk more plainly.

On another occasion, Ms. Williams had been remarkably candid about feelings of loss and her need for other people. Dr. C felt it was important to acknowledge the steps the patient was taking.

Dr. C: You have shown me more of your feelings. You've taken chances by looking at your feelings, looking at things about me and talking with me about them. I think that takes guts. You don't just blow up anymore. You stop, think, try to understand what you're feeling, and then decide what you're going to do.

Helen Jackson had been very intrusive and provocative during the early part of her treatment. In recent sessions, she had been much more thoughtful and open about her emotions.

Dr. S: I feel different with you today. I feel more calm. More relaxed and close to you. Like we have a relationship.

Ms. Jackson nods assent.

Dr. S: I feel this session is much different than a few months ago. I felt that with your barging in and being disruptive, that everything was coming at me at once, that I was being pushed back, that I couldn't think straight. I was anxious. Today, you are more thoughtful, you put your feelings into words. I feel I have room to think, to feel, and I feel closer to you. Also, I feel respect for you more. Not that I didn't respect you before, but I can *feel* it now. I feel like you are someone who has had pain, but who has integrity and value. It was hard to focus on that before with all the antics.

Matters of Style

Prescribing a style for psychotherapy is impossible and undesirable. No doubt, the most helpful psychotherapy approach is a mixture of curiosity about the truth, and respect and affection for the patient. Nevertheless, in work with schizophrenic patients, it may help to consider some stylistic approaches that differ from those commonly used with neurotic or borderline patients. These may expand the horizons of the therapeutic relationship. Of course, this is not to say that each technique is suitable to use with each patient. A playful manner may not be useful at the outset with a patient who complains of despair, inertia, and mental confusion.

    Bluntness. Sometimes, a patient may use the respectful, contained, even temper of the therapist in the service of resistance. He may say or do outrageous things to be provocative. Or, an artificially "professional" tone in the sessions may enable the patient to deny significant emotions. In such situations it can help if the therapist is blunt.

    Ms. Reilley was a hospitalized schizophrenic adolescent who failed at several vocational programs. She had just broken into the office of the occupational therapist and stolen some hospital files, thus risking discharge. She affected an air of nonchalance and brushed off her therapist's effort to focus her on her behavior and its consequences.

Dr. G: You try to be the joker and make everyone laugh while your life goes down the tubes. That's because your life has no value to you.

Ms. R: Huh?

Dr. G: You can't work at a job. And you've told me that no one respects you.

Ms. R: They do so.

Ms. R spits out her gum in the direction of the therapist.

Dr.G: I think you know that spitting at me is not a way for me to respect you more. You don't want to think about it, but you've told me that no one cares what you think and no one cares what you feel. You feel like a zero.

Ms. R: Everything is so screwed up! Everything sucks!

At this point, Ms. Reilley began a more genuine and thoughtful discussion of her feelings of despair.

Play. It may be useful with some patients to find creative ways of communicating and sharing experience. This may involve playing a game together or dispensing with the formality of the setting (for example, taking a walk with the patient, or switching chairs). Encouraging Ms. Thompson to pretend that her therapist was a magician who could grant her wishes is one example. Another, is a role exchange in which the patient playacts the personality and stance of the therapist and vice versa.

Deborah Weiss had been continually complaining of lethargy, mental confusion, and weakness. Several neurological workups were within normal limits, and her sense of torpor was variable and inconsistent over many years. Recently, her physical complaints had become a litany which seemed to kill creativity in sessions. Dr. E suggested that they reverse roles, and Dr. E then began to complain of his tiredness, his fuzzy thinking, and so on. Each time the patient (now acting as Dr. E) would try to open a discussion of Dr. E's feelings or the meaning of his actions, Dr. E slammed the door shut by repeating his somatic complaints. Finally the patient and therapist discussed what this exercise had been like.

Ms. W: I understand now. You're making me see myself better. I'm pushing you away and shutting you down. It's like being constantly pushed away.

Dr. E: Can you see how this might get tiring and make me feel kept at arms' length, and feel like what's the point of working to understand things?

Ms. W: I certainly can.

Chapter 5

Technique in Specific Clinical Situations

THE THERAPEUTIC ALLIANCE AND THE DEGREE OF THERAPIST ACTIVITY

The importance of the interpersonal relationship and the therapeutic alliance was emphasized in chapter 4. Sometimes, however, it is not clear whether making a particular intervention, no matter how reasonable, will strengthen the alliance or alienate the patient. On the one hand schizophrenic patients are enormously sensitive to intrusion and what to them feels like coercion. If they feel invaded or violated, they will flee. Ms. Chen, for example, scrupulously guarded her "personal space." On the other hand, partly because of their use of denial, schizophrenic patients can travel far down the path of self-destruction with little concern, and can quickly bring themselves and their treatments to the brink of collapse. Although they may not acknowledge it consciously, they may leave it to the therapist to act adaptively and help avert disaster. Many circumstances are not clear-cut. The therapist is caught between the Scylla of overactivity and intrusiveness, and the Charybdis of being lulled by the patient's bland denial until suddenly the treatment is destroyed.

Negotiating these waters can be a demanding job. The therapist may feel that it is part of his psychological work to confront and interpret the patient's denial of danger, his use of splitting, and his projection onto the therapist of his own capacity for self-care. For example, Ms. Chen, the teacher, provoked her school principal into firing her by not completing necessary school forms, thus jeopardizing her financial capacity to continue treatment. Nevertheless, she acted as if this was not a subject for discussion and that all somehow would be well. The therapist tried to interpret the patient's use of denial, and pointed out that the treatment would be destroyed if the patient lost her job and could not pay. The patient felt that the therapist was intruding upon her "personal affairs" and declared that it was none of the therapist's business. On the one hand, the therapist cannot simply collude with the patient's denial, while on the other hand, it is, in the end, the patient's life and he must be free to fail. Unfortunately, with schizophrenic patients, the stakes are often very high, and many failures are not easily reversible. Making sound judgments about when simply to listen, when to speak up, and when finally to set limits on the patient's behavior, is a complex and difficult task.

Ms. Chen was suspicious and had numerous ideas of reference at her job. Her relationship with her family was becoming more filled with conflict, and this seemed to put pressure on her rather fragile sense of independence and identity. Frequently, she felt enraged that her autonomy was not respected. During this time, her therapist recommended a consultation with a psychopharmacologist and Ms. Chen reported that she had followed through. This turned out not to be so. Her therapist asked her about the consultation and Ms. Chen became incensed. She admitted that she had not made the appointment, then became evasive and finally accused the therapist of dishonesty. At work, sometime later, she called the assistant principal to her classroom to protect the school against the faculty's dishonesty. The assistant principal called her therapist from school.

When Ms. Chen came for her next session she continued to feel that the troubles at work were part of her "personal space." She denied the emotional, social, and financial danger she was in. Nevertheless, by giving the assistant principal her therapist's telephone number, she implicitly asked the therapist to act as an auxiliary ego.

Despite his chronic psychosis, Mr. DeVito, who was in his midthirties, had worked for fifteen years as an accountant at a bank, had obtained at least two promotions, and, apparently, was well respected at his job. Periodically, Mr. DeVito would become psychotic, and a variety of sexual and aggressive impulses, normally absent, would emerge. His psychoses were usually precipitated by a powerful conflict between a desire to become more independent and develop a more distinct identity, and a wish to become formless and helpless, and thus compel his uncle to intervene and take care of him. Many of his acute episodes were ushered in by concerns about his work, where he felt he was the victim of elaborate plots. He had relatively few friends. When he was not acutely psychotic, he felt that his work was a truly stabilizing force in his life from which he derived a lot of self-esteem. Work was a nidus around which what was clear and distinct in his identity could crystallize.

Mr. DeVito had been more and more agitated and suspicious in recent weeks despite increased dosages of medicine. His chronic delusions about being controlled by a "mafia gangster" were intensifying. He felt increasingly distrustful of his coworkers. He came to a session and announced new plans.

Mr. D: I'm going to leave my job. I think that's the best idea. I have no regrets. I'm going to tell them tomorrow. (Mr. DeVito had already taken several breaks from work, during which he stayed at home and was essentially taken care of by his uncle who lived nearby. Another absence might truly lead to the loss of his job.) Maybe at some point, I'll go back to the bank. But not now. I think maybe I'll open a small business of my own. Anyway, I'm glad I don't have the pressure of going back to the bank.

Mr. DeVito continued in the same vein, with emotional indifference to the consequences of what he was saying. Finally his therapist spoke.

Dr. B: You want to kill off the adult in you, and act as if what you're going to do has no real consequence. I think among other things, you are showing how enraged you are at me and your uncle and aunt, but it comes out in your destroying yourself. But you seem to have no concern about this, as if it doesn't matter. As if your concern for yourself, and your wish to become an adult are locked up in some compartment that doesn't touch you. You say all this in such an offhanded way. As if destroying your adult life is nothing. If you lose your

job, you will have no income, and your uncle will feel
pressured to come in and take care of you. And you
will lose your chance to separate from him and become
an adult. Your goal of growing up and having a relationship with a woman seems to have vanished.

The patient continued to maintain that his actions were no
big deal.

Dr. B: I think your fears about the gangster stand for your
           terror at moving away from your uncle and aunt, which
           you've never done. I think you're furious at them and
           at me about having to become separate. It's easier to
           be taken care of at home. It's as if you want a life of
           leisure with no demands or pressure or risks. Since
           you're not rich, one way to do that is to act like you are
           crippled and frighten your uncle into taking care of
           you. But in doing this your identity as an adult is crum-
           bling. Each day you become more and more like a fea-
           tureless lump. If you have no self, what value would
           your treatment have with me? What goal would we
           have? What would we work on? You're asking me to be
           your doctor and to give you my honest point of view,
           not to watch silently or reassure you while you destroy
           yourself.

    To be sure, this was an uncharacteristically lengthy statement
by Dr. B, but his intention was to interpret the patient's denial
of external social reality, and his use of splitting, which enabled
him to remain unconcerned about what had once been important
wishes for self-sufficiency. Dr. B also wanted to address the patient's wish for an emotional blending with his sister. One might
argue that Dr. B departed from technical neutrality by urging the
patient to take a course of action. From another point of view, Dr.
B was urging him *not* to act precipitously in response to internal
pressure to flee his job. The therapist's goal was not to direct Mr.
DeVito's career choice, but to address the *psychological* processes
that had gathered steam and were threatening to damage his
functioning.

After several sessions such as the one above, the patient, with increased medication, was able to settle down and return to his job.

Clarification, confrontation, and interpretation of splitting, projective identification, denial, and wishes for merger, do not always succeed. The pressure of the patient's inner needs and the impairment of his ego functioning sometimes interfere with his ability to step back, delay, and use concepts to examine what he is doing. In fact, interpretation of primitive defenses can make the patient more evasive and paranoid. These responses alert us to the diagnosis of structural psychosis.

In situations that threaten the patient's physical, social, or financial well-being, and thus, the viability of the treatment, the therapist has no choice but to interpret the use of primitive defenses, even though this may stir up enmity and suspicion in the patient. Certainly, there are less dangerous circumstances in which one can afford to be less therapeutically insistent. To some degree, one's level of activity and persistence can be guided by the patient's subjective capacity to tolerate one's interventions. With sicker patients, one may be tempted to ferret out latent negative transference and primitive defense—to make preemptive strikes, so to speak—so that these processes do not work silently to undermine the treatment (Reich, 1945; Glover, 1955;[1] Kernberg, 1975, 1984). However, such interventions sometimes do intrude upon the patient's freedom to conduct their psychological work in their own way.

Mr. Tilden often jumped from topic to topic during sessions, as if throwing emotional issues overboard, never to be heard of again. There appeared to be few unifying themes. His therapist believed that he used splitting and denial to keep these various aspects of himself disintegrated. She also felt that her confusion must in some way mirror his own. She pointed out that his accounts of himself were usually disjointed, and that he rarely stuck with one topic. This had happened before, and she had not hesitated to interpret his use of splitting, denial, and projection. Now, he responded in a poignant way. He said, simply, that he knew that. He added, "I need to find something to talk about in my

---

[1]Glover (1955) wrote, "The most successful resistances are silent, and it might be said that the sign of their existence, is our unawareness of them" (p. 54).

own way, when I'm ready." The patient and his therapist debated this a bit, but in the end, the therapist thought that maybe Mr. Tindel was right. She relaxed her vigilance concerning the patient's use of primitive defenses and the negative transferences and, in fact, over the following months, the patient did extremely productive work, albeit in a somewhat roundabout way.

In a similar vein, Ms. Chen chided her therapist for what she felt was his excessive activity and concern for the consequences of her behavior. She said, "I don't need a boss to tell me what to do or how to do it. I need someone who will be there to hear me out." She asked in a very ingenuous way if maybe she and the therapist could slow down and let Ms. Chen take more initiative.

On another occasion, Mr. Tilden complained about the therapist's confrontations of his overt and covert aggression.

Mr. T: The way you talk to me makes me feel awful about myself, like I'm a bad, evil person. You say that I hate people. Well, maybe I do. Maybe I do. But I can't take your pushing it in my face all the time. It's too much. I feel like I can't escape it. What do you want me to say? It's true? Okay, it's true. Maybe I'm supposed to be able to handle this being pushed in my face, but I can't. Okay, it's true, I do hate people, but I can't take it's being pushed in my face all the time.

BOUNDARY ISSUES IN THE TREATMENT SETTING

The schizophrenic's problems with the sense of boundary were touched on briefly in chapter 4 and alluded to at the beginning of this chapter. They will be discussed further in chapter 6. A number of primitive defenses appear to contribute to the problem. Rapid cycles of primitive projection and introjection can undermine the distinction between what is self and what is other (Kernberg, 1975, 1984). Defensive fusion of self and object images designed to effect a primal connection (Jacobson, 1964) certainly works against clear definition of boundaries. The boundary between self and other may never have fully matured in the course of development (Schafer, 1968; Loewald, 1980). The deconceptualization of experience and the reperceptualizing or resensationalizing of thought make it difficult for the schizophrenic to discriminate between sensation, perception, thought, feeling, memory, and fantasy, and thus also contribute to the uncertainty about what is inside and what is outside. Scotomatization and denial of perceptions of reality (Freud, 1927, p. 153, n. 2; Jacobson, 1957) undermine the patient's relationship to the external world, and thus contribute to its being confused with the internal.

It is important to keep in mind that the boundary disturbance has an affective as well as a cognitive component. Schizophrenic patients often feel that there is no barrier between the behavior of another person and their own emotional responses. If another person is angry, the patient trembles with fear. If another person commands, the patient feels compelled to obey. There are few inner resources to rely upon for emotional anchorage. It is difficult for the schizophrenic to fend off or insulate himself from external affective influences. The patient feels like a slave to his emotional environment and feels humiliated, impotent, and angry about his capacity to erect an effective barrier to affect. It is unclear whether this emotional porosity is due to a need for a primitive affective unity, a fear of the separateness implied by greater emotional "immunity" from external influence, or is due to a deficit in a neurophysiological stimulus barrier or other factors. Whatever its origins, this porosity probably contributes synergistically to the disturbance in the cognitive margin between inside and outside, and self and other.

The patient's difficulty in discriminating inside from outside, and self from other, can manifest itself very early in treatment. It may make it hard for patient and therapist to engage in a dialogue, or even to occupy the same room. The patient may feel that the therapist is overwhelming him or coercing him or insisting that he submit to the therapist's control. In part because of primitive wishes for fusion, the patient may experience the therapist as intolerably close, so that his sense of separateness is threatened. He may feel that the therapist leaves him no room for a distinct existence, that his heart and soul are being taken over. Or, he may feel that the therapist is interested in him only as an extension of himself, and is not really interested in what the patient actually thinks or feels.

In response to these fears, the patient may try to break off the relationship in order to insure the survival of his own distinct identity. Or, he may try to control the therapist's actions or speech so as to protect himself from intimidation or annihilation. For his part, the therapist may come to feel that he cannot say or do anything, much less anything confrontational or controversial, without the patient becoming enraged or storming out. Thus, the therapist may be tempted to retreat to the position of an observer rather than a participant. Ironically, he may then begin to feel that the patient has come to control *him*, and that his own identity as a therapist is slipping away.

There is no simple solution to this therapeutic predicament. Since from the very outset, the patient may experience conflicts about boundaries, there may be precious little in the way of alliance and goodwill to ease the tensions that develop. One must rely on some combination of countertransference insight, emotional disclosure, tact, humor, inspiration, and patience to find one's way.

A rather long example will, I hope, illustrate this point.

Steven Tilden had just begun his therapy. He came from a family in which he felt that his mother patronized him and was not really interested in what he had to say. He described his father as an extremely conservative and strict man who had to have things his own way. He felt that within the family, his identity had been crushed, and believed that much of his rage stemmed from feeling "squelched."

For several weeks Mr. Tilden seemed very comfortable in sessions and alluded to having a crush on his therapist, but he managed to avoid discussing this in any detail. He missed a few sessions, and then began to talk about his romantic feelings again at the very end of another meeting. He complained that the therapist stopped the session (which she did on time) because she didn't want to hear what he had to say. He was now so angry, he didn't want to talk about the subject anymore.

During the next session, in which he continued to berate his therapist, Dr. T commented that maybe Mr. Tilden wanted to fight with her in order to avoid feeling affection. He promptly became furious and unleashed a stream of invective, complaining that the therapist did not listen and did not care about him. She thought only about herself, and always wanted to bring the focus back to herself. The sessions always focused on what the therapist wanted to discuss, and it was obvious that she didn't give a damn about him. She just wanted to make money and feel like a big shot. He hated her and didn't want to tell her anything. This was all said with great conviction, and a deep feeling of offense.

At this point, the therapist felt roundly criticized. She felt like a little girl who had been scolded, as if she had been bad. She felt sad and guilty. As the session went on, the therapist felt stifled, pent up, inhibited from talking, and demoralized, as if what she had to offer wasn't wanted or needed. She worried that if she didn't say something soon, she would forget what useful ideas she had to offer, and that her sense of therapeutic purpose was evaporating. She felt as if she was simply occupying space in the room.

The therapist encouraged Mr. Tilden to say more, but he was not interested. Finally, not quite knowing what else to do, she shared her personal reactions (detailed above) with the patient. He eyed her with dismay.

Mr. T: You're blaming me again. Everything I do, you find something about it to criticize. You make me feel like I'm a bad person. I *never* get a break, a chance to say what *I* have to say. You always want to do all the talking, I come here to get things off my chest, but you seem to have more of a need to speak than I do. (His face shows great pain.) This is just the same thing that happened at home. I shouldn't have to keep quiet because you have a need to speak.

At this point, the therapist explained her rationale for disclosing her own feelings to the patient. This had been done several times before.

Dr. T: I wasn't trying to criticize you. I told you what I felt because I've found that sometimes the way I'm feeling says something about what you may feel. Like when it's hard for you to keep your thoughts clear. Maybe you feel squelched in some way, then kind of hopeless, and then useless as I did today.

Mr. T: Well, I didn't get that from what you said.

Dr. T: Obviously not.

(Mr. Tilden smiles, and visibly relaxes.)

Mr. T: But you should pay attention to what I was saying. When you're speaking all the time, I don't get a chance. *I* need to get a chance to say what *I* have to. Really, I'm not trying to rebel or give you a hard time. But I have to feel like you're listening to me and that you feel what I'm talking about is important. Otherwise I'll never want to tell you what I'm really feeling inside.

Dr. T: I've thought about this a lot. And when I look within myself I think I was talking in order to say something you should hear. But whether what I said to you was useful or not, I want you to know that I am listening to you about your need to have a chance to say what's on your mind.

Mr. T: What are you feeling now?

Dr. T: More comfortable. More relaxed. And you?

Mr. T: Me too.

It occurred to Dr. T later that Mr. Tilden may have had a need for her to feel squelched and useless not only in order to communicate to her what this experience was like for him, but also to see if she could tolerate these feelings without becoming demoralized or disorganized as he often did.

Another patient, Mr. Stevens, had been talking for about twenty minutes when the therapist made his first comment. Mr. Stevens complained that he was not being given room to talk. The therapist commented that it was as if the "town" were not big enough for the two of them. Either he, the therapist, existed, and Mr. Stevens felt crowded out and annihilated, or Mr. Stevens existed, and the therapist seemed to vanish. It appeared difficult for both of them to exist in their own right, with their separate identities, without one of them feeling erased. Mr. Stevens agreed.

Here is another example. Ms. Chen experienced powerful rages at the people she was closest to, and when under stress, she responded with suspiciousness, and ideas of reference. Her mother had been exceedingly intrusive and destructive of her daughter's autonomy. Ms. Chen had missed one recent session, and now asked if she and the therapist could reduce the frequency of their sessions. Among other things, the therapist asked Ms. Chen about her feelings toward him. The patient seemed upset and said that she did not want to talk about the relationship. The therapist asked her why not. Ms. Chen answered that the more they talked about their relationship, the more she would be burdened, and the more she would have to worry about the therapist. Whenever the therapist asked her about her personal feelings toward her, Ms. Chen felt as if a dentist were probing at her skull rather than her mouth with an instrument.

Ms. Chen's fears illustrate how fragile was her grasp of her own separateness. Her worries also demonstrate the intimate connection between boundary disturbances and disturbances of identity. She continually tried to shore up the boundary between herself and her therapist because she feared that otherwise, her life and the therapist's would begin to run together like watercolors. She would feel prodded and poked like a research specimen. She also feared that the therapist would change the shape of her body. Ms. Chen had used the image of her body shape before, and it seemed to be a metaphor for her sense of identity. If patient and therapist got too close, the therapist would have undue influence over her, she felt, and could alter her according to her will. Ms. Chen's fear of influence seems to be a good example of the *affective* boundary disturbance mentioned at the outset of this chapter.

THE EXPERIENCE OF EMPTINESS AND DEADNESS AND ITS IMPACT ON THE THERAPIST'S CAPACITY TO LISTEN

Often, if not invariably, schizophrenic patients feel empty and dead. We can understand this in several ways. Emotions often produce such pain or fear that patients try to protect themselves against affects of any kind (Eissler, 1953b, 1954; Will, 1975; Searles, 1979, p. 16).

Some patients seem to distinguish between emptiness and deadness. Phenomenologically, emptiness seems to refer to a state of "missing" something of which they are only dimly aware. It is very painful and exerts a persistent pressure. Patients who describe this kind of emptiness are motivated to remove this state with some form of input, satisfaction, or distraction. In contrast, patients who feel dead inside, seem not so much anguished as apathetic. They are not so much searching for something that will pleasantly fill them up, or relieve an inner gnawing, as they are mechanically going through the motions without desire. They are indifferent to everything.

Both the experience of emptiness and deadness can play a central role in the emotional lives of schizophrenic patients.

Mr. DeVito referred to his emotional life as a "desolate valley where no one ever sets foot." If someone did appear, the patient would feel unnatural and grotesque next to a person who was "real." His inner life, he said, felt like a gray dungeon.

Ms. Weiss said, "I am barren. There is nothing inside to give to anyone."

Ms. Chen disclosed, "I feel like a forest after a fire, with no trees. It needs people to care for it, to fertilize, plow, and plant trees so there can be some life." Later, she added, "Sometimes in my imagination, I see a photograph of my body which is crumpled and torn into bits."

Ms. Williams, a tough, pragmatic young woman, not given to lyrical abstractions, self-disclosure, or hyperbole, said, "At times it's like I am a huge expanse of nothing. I don't feel human when I'm all alone."

A number of patients referred to a sense of deadness. Both Mr. DeVito and Ms. Weiss referred to themselves as "dead heads." Ms. Weiss commented that her emotions were "dead and buried." Mr. Sands, another schizophrenic patient, reported, "Nothing seems like it's worth doing. Everything just seems empty. I have nothing to talk about."

The etiology of these patients' feelings of emptiness and deadness is unclear. Psychologically, patients may defend themselves against tormenting affects by shutting down their emotional reactivity. Ms. Williams stated, "The feeling of missing people is torture, not physical torture, but mental torture." Mr. DeVito, who complained that his feeling of emptiness was like having "pieces of iron" in his stomach, said, "I'd rather have iron than feel desperate and alone." These defenses may lead to a shut down of feeling or desire or both, and, thus, progressively to emptiness and then deadness.

Or, the sense of emptiness may express a painful, inescapable, gnawing hunger for soothing, relief, and spirit-quickening contact. The feeling may express a structuralized and chronic emotional position, or a more transient contemporary experience.

Often, there is no active intervention which will directly relieve these patients of the pain, hopelessness, futility, or nihilism that arise from feeling empty or dead. Straightforward encouragement may be temporarily soothing, but frequently it does little to change the patient's chronic inner experience.

Nevertheless, I include the description of emptiness in this chapter on technique because it does require a specific and very difficult technical response: listening. To listen to the patient talk about his inner hollowness, his feeling of being inhuman, his humiliating envy of the therapist for having all the patient himself wishes to have, is hard to tolerate. In this sense, these patients are not emotionally impoverished. If one marks the depth of the patient's emotional life by the depth of poignant pain it can induce in the therapist, then these patients' emotions run frighteningly deep. It is not easy to sit with someone, encourage him to take off his emotional shirt, and then stare at his gaping affective wounds. No doubt this is part of why the practice of doing psychotherapy with schizophrenic patients has not inspired more enthusiasm. Approaching schizophrenic patients from a pharmacological, biological, or learning theory perspective, as valid and useful as these avenues are, may spare the clinician from some of the deepest reaches of countertransference pain.

In order to help the patient with feelings of emptiness and deadness, the clinician must be willing to tolerate the stirring up of similar feelings in himself via emotional induction. He must also be willing to feel his own versions of emptiness, nihilism, deadness, hopelessness, and envy. The patient *may* feel less isolated, excommunicated, and alien if he feels that the therapist is comprehending his inner experience, and that there is common ground between him and the clinician (Sullivan, 1953).[2] The patient will certainly *not* feel differently if the therapist cannot receive these disturbing and intense feelings into his heart. I am not saying that the therapist should suffer in the same way the patient does. Even if it were possible, that would lead to dysfunction and is based on a false premise of symbiotic cure. But to

---

[2]Sullivan wrote, "Everyone is much more simply human than otherwise" (1953, p. 32). He referred to this as the "one-genus hypothesis."

avoid emotions which are induced by the patient is to lose an essential compass in guiding the therapeutic work. It is also, perhaps, to lose an opportunity to send a crucial signal to the patient that the therapist cares enough to stand by him in his pain.

PRESSURED SPEECH AND LOOSENESS OF ASSOCIATION

In many of the examples I have cited so far, the patients have spoken relatively coherently, even if angrily, contemptuously, or irrationally. Of course, this does not always happen, and many schizophrenic patients demonstrate looseness of association, tangentiality, and circumstantiality. Since verbal psychotherapy depends on the patient telling a reasonably coherent story, what does one do?

In my experience, it has been helpful to apply the techniques of naming and enlargement to the patient's bizarre productions. Often, the therapist must first explain to the patient why he, the therapist, is interrupting: that the therapist is taking the patient's use of words *very* seriously, that the patient is going too quickly, or jumping too fast for the therapist to follow. The patient is encouraged to slow down, take one idea at a time, and explain in great detail precisely what he means.

Some patients are able rather quickly to make use of this advice. They are able, in fact, to slow down, and although further clarification is necessary, their story becomes much more comprehensible.

Other patients do not benefit so quickly. In these cases, it is worthwhile to inquire whether the patient understands why the therapist is saying that his remarks are hard to follow. The patient's idiosyncratic speech may reflect a psychotic incapacity to empathize with the social criteria of reality (Kernberg, 1975, 1984). The patient may not understand how another person reacts to this behavior. If this is so, it may be helpful to underscore how difficult it is to follow him, and to suggest that he speak more slowly, more clearly, and with fewer sudden leaps of content.

Or, the patient may be motivated to be incoherent. Recall Ms. Williams who said that she spoke incoherently at activities therapy because she did not want others to know what she was feeling. Words are powerful tools which can help send messages about inner states from one subjectivity to another, but they also can be used to mislead, deceive, evade, hide, and obscure. One may need to examine with the patient whether he wants or does not want the therapist to understand him. If he does not, it is important to know more about why not. It may be useful to make a joint agreement about which subjects the patient feels comfortable discussing, and which, for now, at least, he does not.

Ms. Jackson, a black woman in her late twenties, began her session by talking rapidly. She jumped from one subject to another. In the course of about five minutes, she talked about how she missed her boyfriend, then about how they attended a party, then about how it was when she was living with her aunt, then about her sister's work as a teacher. The transitions were abrupt, and while her therapist assumed these subjects were connected, and could make up connections to fit, the rush of topics seemed like a jumble.

Dr. S: I am sorry to stop you, but you started by talking about your boyfriend, and ended up talking about your sister being a teacher. How did you make that jump?

           Ms. Jackson repeated a similarly pressured, obscure sequence.

Dr. S: Again, I'm sorry to stop you, but you're talking about one thing and then go on to several others. Can you see that it would be hard for me to follow you along?
Ms. J: Yes. I do know what you mean. I think I want to talk about my boyfriend.

Ms. Jackson proceeded to talk about her boyfriend in a way that the therapist could follow.

Dorothy Hunt was a young woman who had florid psychotic symptoms for many years. She was grossly delusional, had paranoid ideas, ideas of reference, auditory hallucinations, and inappropriate affect. She had no friends.

Ms. H: I want to be a farmer and I want to live in a commune because the air in the day hospital is so bad, I can't breathe it. And everyone knows you can't be healthy if the air is no good. The air you breathe makes you what you are. Don't you think?

Dr. U: From what I can tell farming and good air are very important to you.

Ms. H: Well, yes. Anyway that's what the spirits are making me feel. They influence me from the stove.

Dr. U: You're telling me that spirits influence you from the stove?

Ms. H: Uh huh. But I never really made any friends when I lived with my grandfather.

Dr. U: I'm going to interrupt you. It's not because I'm not interested in what you're saying, but because I take each of your words very seriously. I want to make sure I understand each of them.

Ms. H: My aunt wants me to call her every day and . . .

Dr. U: You know, I'm sure what you're saying is important. And I want to ask you more about it in a little while. But, first, I want to make sure I understand what you were saying about the spirits. That seems important to you since you've brought it up several times today. Do they live there? Are they there all the time? How did they get there? How do they know about you, and why do you think they are interested in you? (The day before, the patient and therapist had begun to discuss the spirits.)

Ms. H: You know, I was watching TV, and an old episode of "Dragnet" came on and . . .

Dr. U: Can you see how I might think that you are changing the subject?

Ms. H: I guess I did.

The doctor and patient finally were able to discuss the spirits in a less haphazard, more comprehensible way.

The same patient, several months later, had just come from an interview at a day program.

Dr. U: How did it go?

Ms. H: They are all talking about me. Like they know something about me. There was something in the air, like drugs. Or maybe some kind of poison. You know, I like to take a shower at least twice a day. To have a fresh smell. I wonder if my grandfather remembers that I stole money from him.

Dr. U: You know, I'm not sure I understand. You've talked about so many subjects, it's hard for me to keep them straight. When I stop you it's so that I can really try to understand each of the ideas you're telling me about, each of the words you use. Otherwise it would be like you're talking to the wall. Maybe you don't really *want* me to understand you, like when someone uses a secret code. But if you do want me to know what you're saying, you need to slow down. And I'll probably need to stop you and ask more questions.

Ms. H: I see your point.

Ms. Bender was a 45-year-old woman who was grossly dishevelled, had chronic auditory hallucinations and somatic delusions, and who lived in a supervised residence. She had not worked in years, and had no friends. She had lived with a roommate in a supervised residence. This relationship developed into perhaps the deepest friendship she had ever experienced. She began the session in the following way:

Ms. B: My friendship was like a chocolate cake.

Dr. M: How do you mean?

There was a long pause.

Dr. M: I think that comparing your friendship to a cake probably has a lot of meaning. I want to try as best I can to understand what you're trying to say. How was it that your friendship was like a chocolate cake?

Ms. B: When I came back to the apartment, Sandra and I would listen to music together. (Pause). The feeling was good.

Dr. M: So, looking back on the times you were with Sandra, listening to music, there was a particularly good feeling.

Silence.

Dr. M: And the picture of the chocolate cake? If I think of chocolate cake, I get a picture of something sweet, special, and delightful.

Ms. B: Our friendship was barren and cozy.
Dr. M: Can you tell me some more about the barren part?

Ms. Bender looked pained and sad. After a long time she spoke.

Ms. B: Dr. M, certain things are impediments. I think I've lost my breath for today.
Dr. M: If you don't want to go on with a subject, please let me know. We don't have to continue with this right now if you're not ready to talk about it. Just let me know if you don't want to talk about something, and we'll wait for a time that you feel more able to. All you have to say is: "I don't want to talk about that right now." I don't want to talk about anything which is uncomfortable for you when you're not ready or don't want to.

The approach to pressured speech and looseness of association that I have described addresses the relationship between the speaker and the listener. It assumes that even if the patient is communicating idiosyncratically, that there remains a nonpsychotic part of his personality. This nonpsychotic part is capable of understanding that he is either not making the effort to translate his inner experience into conventional and public symbols (words), or is failing in that effort. This approach addresses the *process* of communication, rather than the content per se, so that a more reliable form of exchange can occur, and the clinician is not left, session after session, to perform miracles of comprehension.

There is another approach, which may be useful from time to time, and that is to treat the patient's words as word conglomerates, not sentences. Freud (1900) described how the manifest dream text was actually a conglomerate, a patchwork of symbols and signs which had no *conceptual* relation to one another (except that added by secondary revision). The elements were related not by *conceptual* or *logical* association, but by associations based on contiguity in time, place, sound, and so on. The speech of schizophrenics, similarly, consists of conglomerates of ideas, symbols, and associations, and as the patient talks a kind of background music may emerge. Ideas and affects related to certain themes may appear. The theme of Ms. Bender's cake metaphor was intimacy and loss. Ms. Bender and Dr. M had many more conversations which were much more opaque than the one described above, and which would be much too long to quote in full. They required many slowings-down, much naming and enlargement, and very often yielded themes related to sadness, loss, and loneliness. As mentioned above, however, even when she and Dr. M were able to understand the meanings behind her statements, the method of communicating and translating remained problematic.

HALLUCINATIONS AND DELUSIONS

Hallucinations

The approach to the patient who has hallucinations is not markedly different from the patient who has looseness of associations. Assuming one had already used neuroleptic medicine in optimal doses, one wants to address the use to which hallucination is put, as well as the content. Patients often use hallucinations as alternatives to conceptual forms of communication, both to others and to themselves. Searles wrote, "In general, and to a high degree, schizophrenic patients experience inner emotions not as such, but rather as distorted perceptions of the outside world" (1979, p. 13). In other words, the patient defends himself from too poignant, too frightening, or painful emotions by taking them out of the realm of the "inner life," and out of a form (concepts) which convey their meanings and connection to other meanings. Such richness and echoing of meaning is simply too painful or overwhelming. Emotions are deflated, deconceptualized, desymbolized, and finally sensualized and perceptualized. The patient does not feel sad, but has the sensation that his heart is heavy and literally sinking in his chest (e.g., Mr. DeVito). The patient does not feel angry at his boss, but rather experiences heat in his chest (e.g., Mr. DeVito). The patient does not feel pressured by his therapist, but has the sensation of a dental instrument pushing on her skull (e.g., Ms. Chen).

In order to understand what lies behind the hallucination psychologically, one must explore it using naming and enlargement. The goal is to return the emotional and conceptual associations which have been squeezed out of the patient's inner life. In illness, surplus emotional meaning infuses the patient's physical sensations, making them bizarre and uncanny (Bion, 1956). If the therapist explores these sensations with the patient, and asks him all that comes to his mind about them, exactly what they feel like, where they occur, and what thoughts or feelings accompany them, feelings and meanings may begin to seep into the patient's account.

As noted before, Ms. Bender came for her session, and Dr. M asked her what had led to her hospitalization. She evaded the question and went on to discuss other things in a desultory way. Dr. M led her back to the topic of her hospitalization, and she then reported seeing an object which looked like sandpaper near Dr. M's chair. Dr. M asked her what this looked like and what it made her think of. She described the appearance as rough and abrasive. Finally, she said, "Like the appearance of someone who is irritating and pushy." The patient and therapist then talked about her dislike of Dr. M's persistent questioning about her family.

Delusions

Obviously, delusions are complex phenomena. They may be connected to perceptual distortions such as hallucinations. One may hear *sounds* or voices coming from the refrigerator; that is a hallucination. To develop the related *belief* that this means that people live in the refrigerator, is a delusion. A delusion is a belief, not consensually validated, that is maintained with a certainty. If the patient is not certain about his belief, if he entertains some doubt, we may call this an overvalued idea, and conclude that his reality testing remains intact.

Psychologically, delusions come about because of the interaction of the patient's wishes with his perceptions and concepts about what is real. Strengthening or weakening of either element can alter the balance of forces and result in either more realistic or less realistic beliefs. If the patient uses the defense of denial and blocks out the awareness of large portions of external reality, then conviction about his fantasied version of that reality is given freer license. If the individual's wishful needs to maintain a particular belief grow powerful, then even if the functioning of his ego is usually intact, his need may overwhelm his powers of observation. If, for example, one is captured and held hostage, one may defensively come to believe in the righteousness of one's captor's cause.

Delusion formation may be seen as closely related to the process of forming and telling lies. We develop a lie, an altered version of reality, for the consumption of those around us, because it serves our interests. Often, these lies serve our emotional needs. While a lie may at first be the product of a conscious, intentional act, over the passage of time the circumstances of its origins may fade in memory, and the emotional comfort it gives may be so compelling that it acquires an affective *feeling* of reality. It may sometimes be a rather short step to develop a *cognitive* conviction as well.

Superego functioning, no doubt, plays an important role in this process. Hartmann (1953, pp. 200–203) has discussed the role of superego functioning in the testing of reality. One's "moral" allegiance to truth telling (and thinking for that matter) which develops in the context of object relations within the family, may affect one's willingness or unwillingness to "modify" truths for defensive purposes.

In any case, with patients who present delusions, it is valuable to determine whether they unequivocally believe in the distortion they report. When confronted with contradictions in their stories, or with the illogic or lack of consensual validation of what they assert, patients may acknowledge that, perhaps, their belief is not so. In this case, the patient is not psychotic, at least so far as this particular belief is concerned. He may, in fact, simply be lying. He may be presenting what appears to be a delusional belief, ultimately knowing it to be untrue, for ulterior, and perhaps manipulative reasons.

To complicate this further, we may theoretically believe that there is always a nonpsychotic part of the patient's personality. If this is so, then there remains a part of the psychotic patient's mind that is aware that his delusional belief is false. The difference between delusion and lie then hangs on how integrated or conscious this "nonpsychotic" portion is, or is not. Evaluating this can be tricky indeed.

In any event, the approach to the patient with delusions is complicated. Mostly, it serves no purpose to confront the patient with "the truth." The patient has developed his distortion over time for powerful reasons, not easily swept away by common sense. Two procedures are useful. First, it is important to understand the emotions that are connected to the delusion. We then may be able to grasp the context in which the delusional belief occurs, and what function it serves in the patient's psychic economy. Second, the clinician can tactfully inquire about how the patient understands the relation between this (delusional) belief and other beliefs of his which seem to contradict it. This is *not* done to coerce the patient's agreement with convention, but to map out the boundaries of the distortion and, if possible, help the patient become aware of his own potential for doubt.

Mr. DeVito had once again come to fear being taken over by the "gangster." He believed that the head of an organized crime family somehow lived in his heart. The gangster would eventually take over his mind, leading to terrible consequences. Eventually, everyone would be destroyed.

Increasingly, Mr. DeVito felt the influence of the gangster in his heart and was becoming suspicious of his colleagues at the bank.

Mr. D: The gangster is getting stronger.
Dr. B: How do you know?
Mr. D: Two clerks at the bank told me so.
Dr. B: Why would you believe them?
Mr. D: When I have confidence in someone, I tend to believe them.
Dr. B: But, if I told you that you were Cary Grant, you'd think something was fishy.
Mr. D: (Laughing.) That's true.
Dr. B: Well, I guess what I don't understand is why you'd put stock in what these two clerks have to say. You hardly even know them, much less have reason to trust them.
Mr. D: I'm not sure.

After some more discussion, Mr. DeVito continued.

Mr. D: I'm ready to stand up to the gangster now. I know if you're honest and good, it gives you strength.

Dr. B: So being honest and good gives you strength to stand up to the gangster. What has made you believe more in your honesty and goodness?

Mr. D: Before I believed all the rumors and lies about me.

Dr. B: Are you saying that when other people don't believe in you that it weakens your own faith in yourself?

Mr. D: Definitely.

Dr. B: Can you give me an example of how other people's lack of faith weakened you?

Mr. D: Yes, my uncle sometimes tells me I'm sick, and that I shouldn't try to do too much for myself. When he says things like that I feel why bother trying. What's the point?

Dr. B: Why do you think you let your uncle's ideas influence you so much?

Mr. D: I don't know. It's important to me that he likes me.

Dr. B: What you're saying is that because you want him to approve of you, you're willing to change your opinion about yourself.

Mr. D: Yes.

Mr. DeVito went on to talk about how he first came to believe that a gangster lived in his heart. He said he was in an Italian restaurant when he heard a voice, like when you hear your own thoughts. Dr. B asked if the voice was inside or outside his head. Outside, he said. He then thought he heard a waiter and waitress talking about how organized crime would take over everything. These thoughts are *not mine*, he thought.

Dr. B. took a moment to explain the reason for his questions.

Dr. B: I want to be clear. I am *not* trying to influence your beliefs about the gangster. I want to know more about how your ideas and feelings connect with each other, and how your beliefs about the gangster have become so strong.

At another point, Mr. DeVito was again fearful of the influence of the gangster. He had just returned from the hospital where he had cardiac angiography. His doctors had shown him some of the X ray films of his heart. Dr. B asked if the X rays and dye studies had shown the presence of the gangster. Patient and therapist discussed the ins and outs of this. Mr. DeVito speculated that the gangster somehow wouldn't show up on the X rays. The therapist pointed out that if he were a miniature person as the patient had maintained, the gangster's bones would appear as densities on the films. Dr. B did not push this too far, and certainly did not try to "prove" that Mr. DeVito's ideas were irrational. Dr. B touched on this subject simply to explore the boundaries of the patient's ideas, and also, to add a quantum of uncertainty to a yet modest, but developing sense of doubt in the patient's mind.

It may be useful to acknowledge explicitly to the patient that patient and therapist have two very different views of reality. It is not necessary for the therapeutic work that both therapist and patient agree fully with each other, even about matters of "fact." The therapist can say that it is not his intent to pressure the patient to agree with his point of view, and that he hopes the patient and he can find a way to work together, and respect one another, even while important questions remain undecided.

It can happen that as time goes on, pieces and chunks of past experience and fantasy become more clear, giving at least some picture of how a delusion may have been formed from its building blocks. It turned out that when Mr. DeVito was 7 years old, his 9-year-old sister became ill and the family's attention focused upon her needs. The illness lasted several years and Mr. DeVito felt left out, overlooked, and resentful. He recalled how his father had boxed with him as a child, and accidentally delivered a powerful blow to his chest, leaving the boy with "an aching feeling in my heart." When he was a child, his father's best friend, also a boxer, told him lurid stories about Cosa Nostra chiefs who exerted control and power over the lives of others in his native Sicily. In his current life, Mr. DeVito feels that his uncle is too much a part of his life, and has too much influence over him.

Now, of course, much of this history given by the patient might have been confabulated. Even if it were not, to present the patient with an intellectual solution to the cognitive riddle which his delusion presented, would not help much. The patient does not adhere to the delusion in the present because of faulty memory, or an inadequate capacity to translate symbols. There are powerful contemporaneous as well as historical motives which compel belief. But it may be helpful, as an addition to the general work, to trace the evolution of an idea with the patient. The patient's capacity for intellectual mastery can be a useful ally.

IDEAS OF REFERENCE

Ideas of reference can stir up torment in schizophrenic patients. The patient may believe that those around him are mocking him, ridiculing him, sneering at him, or betraying him. The social environment becomes a dense misty wood in which the patient's sense of safety and self-esteem can be ambushed without warning. Usually, such ideas are associated with vigilance, paranoid ideas, and guardedness.

Ideas of reference are often accompanied by the feeling that there is extra meaning in one's environment. Things do not happen either coincidentally or distinct from a meaningful connection to oneself. Often, a patient believes that events contain elliptical references in word or deed to himself. The people around the patient will not come out and say directly what they mean. They leave signs, suggestions, and hints.

My impression is that the presence of ideas of reference is associated with a significant disturbance of self-esteem and the sense of boundary. The patient often has an agonizing sense of worthlessness, smallness, oddness, or badness. He believes that he has no clothes to conceal these disfigurements of his value, and that his own impression of himself is virtual public knowledge. The uncertainty and tension this creates is like a brooding creature, ready to attack. The patient may act to resolve his disturbing doubts by confronting others about their opinions, beliefs, actions, or comments to him in order to either reassure himself that they have not been malicious, or to clarify that they have. All this may be done in an effort to master terrible anxiety. This solution, which is usually far out of step with social reality, of course, makes matters worse. The patient often *does* then become the object of notice, curiosity, and hushed discussion.

What seems to add to the growth of ideas of reference is the patient's own tendency himself to communicate in indirect, cryptic ways. He may lock his door to show that he does not want to be interfered with. He may come uninvited to a work meeting to express his hurt and anger about not having been invited to an unrelated gathering. He may act provocatively in psychotherapy, bringing limit-setting controls upon himself, instead of expressing his fear that he will choke his therapist.

Cathy Chen, the woman who was so prone to explosions of rage, had a new neighbor where she lived. Ms. Chen felt that this man was very intrusive. The newcomer inquired where Ms. Chen had lived previously, what she did for a living, and so on, which made Ms. Chen suspicious and guarded. She felt that the man was loud and boisterous. All this made her angry.

In response, Ms. Chen put a note in her neighbors' mailboxes which informed them that all new tenants had to sit on the board of a major charitable organization in order to join the tenants' association.

As best her therapist could tell, the translation of this message was: "You know who you are. You are an uncouth, uncivilized low life. It is not *my* credentials that should be inspected. *Your* qualifications will be scrutinized. If you want to associate with me, you'd better change your ways."

Ms. Chen made no effort to speak to her neighbor directly, or to find some more specific, limited, and neutral way to express her unhappiness and persuade her neighbor to be more respectful of her privacy. Because of her own poor social skills, because of her fear of retaliation, or the danger of her own anger getting out of control, or because of her fear that she would be exposed as inadequate, she did not communicate directly with the new neighbor. Instead, she chose to aim a cryptic message at a diffuse target. The therapist's impression was that Ms. Chen believed that others felt and communicated as she did. For her, the emotional airwaves were crammed with cryptic messages about others and about herself.

Of course, as with many schizophrenic phenomena, there is a grain of truth in this belief. We all communicate indirectly some of the time both unintentionally and intentionally. Our facial expressions, tone of voice, and behavior reveal eminently decipherable messages that sometimes we do not intend to send. And we also sometimes choose not to be explicit with our intended audience: we often hint, imply, and give clues. The tendency to scan for hidden meanings, and to send coded messages like Ms. Chen, is not wholly alien to normal functioning. But for a patient with ideas of reference, what one might call the "diplomatic" function is disturbed. Such a patient finds it hard to judge what is an intentional and what is an unintentional communication. He cannot gauge what the other person knows and does not know about the message he (the other person) is sending. He cannot judge, for example, how he should react when he correctly picks up unconscious resentment on the part of another. Should this be considered part of life's normal ups and downs, and passed over unless it persists? Or, should he feel attacked, and protect his safety and honor with a counteroffensive, or by breaking off the relationship entirely? Because the sense of boundary of these patients is disturbed, and because their needs for contact, safety, and esteem are so urgent, these questions cannot be considered calmly and cooly, but seem to call for immediate and decisive action.

Ms. Bennet was leaving her favorite bakery. Traffic was bad due to a water main break. The saleswoman remarked, "Watch out for the traffic on 96th Street, Ms. Bennet. It's pretty bad." The patient was furious. Who did this person think she is? Ms. Bennet telephoned the owner and threatened to contact the Better Business Bureau if this happened again. Several weeks later, the patient noticed that she had been overcharged on a utility bill. She wondered whether the saleswoman somehow had a hand in this and was retaliating against her for her phone call.

Part of what may contribute to the feeling of extra meaning in the environment, is the disturbance in the patient's sense of distinct identity. For reasons discussed earlier (primitive projection, fusion of self and object images, inability to identify and conceptualize affects, etc.) the patient's sense of his own identity is diffuse and confusing. He is frequently unclear about his own motives and principles, and is equally bewildered about those of others. It is as if he has been placed in a Byzantine court, and has no idea what the various bowings and gestures signify.

Combining deconceptualization with the absence of empathy for what is customary, Ms. Chen reported that her uncle once advised her not to let men "take her to the cleaners." It so happened that Ms. Chen's boyfriend one night offered to help her with her laundry. Was this okay? Is this what her uncle had warned against?

PARANOIA

The psychotherapy of paranoid patients is filled with treacherous pitfalls. Certain patients may have paranoid experiences which are limited to the transference and do not deteriorate into frank psychosis. They are able to maintain an image of the therapist which is not completely corrupted by their suspiciousness and can continue to depend on him in an inappropriate way. They have the capacity to doubt a developing feeling of certainty which goes along with their paranoid view, and thus, strictly speaking, their beliefs can be considered "overvalued ideas."

Other patients who are not necessarily structurally psychotic may experience "transference psychoses" (Searles, 1965; Kernberg, 1975, 1984) and develop suspicious delusions which are limited to the psychotherapy setting. Still another group of patients are delusionally paranoid both within the treatment, and in the outside world.

Working with patients who are hostile and suspicious is, perhaps, the psychotherapist's most taxing challenge. Such patients often attack the setting, the procedure, and the therapist with alarming viciousness, exhausting persistence, and considerable destructive skill. Kernberg (1984) has identified one such group of patients with borderline structure as having "malignant narcissism." Whether they are structurally borderline or psychotic, these patients often are extremely vulnerable to a painful sense of worthlessness, have a feeling of a "shattering" of the sense of self, and need to assign rigid roles to others in the service of managing their self-feeling. They also have a capacity for intense rage, destructiveness, and revenge when they feel they have been "crossed." Disappointment and a feeling of betrayal in the transference may lead to attacks on the therapist or a precipitous rupture of the therapeutic relationship.

There are no ready solutions for approaching the therapeutic dilemmas which these patients present. Frequently, these patients are filled with rage, and this rage and the defenses against it infiltrate the transference and extratransference object relations. Devaluation, contempt, and hostile withdrawal make it very difficult for these patients to admire, trust, and rely on anyone, and this complicates their lives in and out of treatment. They often are unable to get emotional nourishment or soothing from relationships, and this simply reinforces their sense of deprivation and isolation, and increases their envy and rage. The cycle of unfulfilled need, anger, devaluation, withdrawal, and further unfulfilled need repeats itself. When they do not withdraw outright from interpersonal contact, they regard attempts to engage them as dangerous intrusions which can leave them vulnerable to tantalization, seductive manipulation, exploitation, or disguised attack. The therapist who wishes to make contact with such a patient sometimes feels he must maintain an almost saintly level of integrity in order to disabuse the patient of his suspicions. Needless to say, this is not possible.

The vicious cycle described above often will not change of its own accord. The therapist may feel it necessary to interpret primitive defenses such as devaluation, projective identification, splitting, denial, and omnipotent control which underlie it (Kernberg, 1975). Theoretically this is a sound approach, and clinically it is often extremely useful. But unlike work with many borderline patients, such interpretations do not necessarily reduce the use of these defenses (Kernberg, 1975, 1984). Patients with psychotic structure may become more enraged, more paranoid, more confused, or more psychotic.

The alternative course—listening to the patient's paranoid or hostile communication without interpreting aggression systematically—has its pitfalls as well. While some advocate such an approach for narcissistic personality disorder and for schizophrenia (Spotnitz, 1969), this path is problematic. Silence may be interpreted by the patient either as tacit agreement with the patient's devaluation, or acquiescence with his destruction of what is good in the therapeutic relationship. If the image of the therapist is sufficiently degraded, the patient may feel a sense of triumph, but will not be able to depend upon the clinician for the help he needs.

Much of the debate surrounding the treatment of narcissistic personality focuses upon the choice between interpreting primitive defenses on the one hand, and and avoiding confrontation in an effort to provide a benign "mirror" for the patient to use as he needs. Kernberg (1984) recommends the interpretation of primitive defenses and the "grandiose self" in an effort to enable the patient to realistically depend on the therapist. By contrast, Kohut (1971) recommends little initial activity in order to allow narcissistic transferences to build and deepen. Kohut's belief is that gradually the patient himself will come to recognize the defensive and maladaptive nature of his object relations.

Whatever may be the case in the treatment of patients with narcissistic personality disorder, one may not have the luxury of waiting with paranoid patients, especially those with psychotic structure. The transference of these patients does not often lead to spontaneous resolution via insight, and while paranoid trends may appear to vanish on their own, in fact they may simply go underground to reappear at another time. There are some who recommend trying to "merge as completely as possible into the friendly expanses surrounding the patient" (Balint, 1959, p. 97) in treating schizophrenics, but there is often precious little friendly space to blend into when working with patients who are paranoid.

Ms. Chen had been in treatment for several years and had been doing well. However, over the course of about a month she became increasingly suspicious. She got into altercations with her fellow teachers, feeling that the public address system at her job was being used to disseminate hostile messages about her. Finally, she called the assistant principal to her classroom to report accusations against her colleagues, and the administrator, in turn, called her therapist, Dr. N. When she met next with Dr. N, Ms. Chen appeared haggard and tense. She had not consulted with a psychopharmacologist as Dr. N had recommended. When Dr. N asked her about what had happened at school, Ms. Chen tensed further and felt that the therapist was intruding. She said she felt as if there was a "dental instrument pushing on my skull." Ms. Chen had precipitated a crisis which created all kinds of dangers for her, both social and financial. While she implicitly was asking the therapist to help by giving the assistant principal her telephone number, she bristled at Dr. N's request for details and gave the impression that she was taking care of things just fine on her own. She said, "I don't pay you to teach me things; I pay you to listen." Essentially, she denied the call for help implied in the crisis she had created. She was furious with Dr. N for not sharing her own view of reality. At this point, she could not tolerate that there could be two very different, incompatible views of what was real. If Dr. N did not see the world the way she did, it seemed, then Dr. N was part of the problem, and was against her.

During her meeting with Ms. Chen, Dr. N tried both to obtain the details about what had happened, and also to point out that although she and the patient saw the world very differently, this did not necessarily mean they could not work together. Dr. N also pointed out how furious Ms. Chen was, and how that made it difficult for her to trust others, including the therapist. After a few more meetings, the patient stopped coming to her sessions.

The therapist later found out from her relatives that the patient had been extremely upset because her boyfriend had criticized her for forgetting to buy concert tickets. The patient became massively enraged, and then withdrawn.

Mr. Martin was a 25-year-old accountant who had never been hospitalized or overtly psychotic. He did have at least one and possibly two first-degree relatives who were schizophrenic. On the surface, he appeared to be a man with narcissistic personality disorder. He depended on others inordinately for his self-esteem, and became enraged when he was disappointed. There was a haughty quality to him, and his idealization of others was often followed by bitter devaluation and contempt. He used splitting and projective identification prominently as defenses. His superego functioning was inconsistent, and while he excoriated others for dishonesty and disloyalty to him, he rationalized his own dishonesties and petty thefts (he periodically shoplifted). He had little tolerance for guilt, and usually projected responsibility for destructiveness onto others, maintaining an image of himself as a victim.

He appeared to relate to the therapist in the transference as both confirmer of his ideas and values, and as an ally against those who did not understand him. As long as the therapist did not question his feelings or behavior, he saw her in a positive light. When the therapist asked about incidents in which he had become suspiciously hostile, or interpreted his primitive defenses, he became guarded and angry.

Mr. Martin's symptoms were exacerbated when his girl friend of several years left to take a job in another city. He became agitated and suspicious. He was both destructively hostile and clinging to this woman at the same time. He visited her at work to excoriate her. Despite his repeated criticisms, he could not refrain from making some kind of contact. He felt both furious and tormented for weeks.

Gradually, his behavior deteriorated. He got into conflicts with the law (for shoplifting and disturbing the peace) and came to several sessions high on drugs. The therapist, Dr. R, pointed out the self-destructive nature of his behavior, and interpreted his use of splitting and projective deidentification. She raised the question of whether his self-destructive behavior was a criticism of his girl friend and herself for not caring for him enough. The patient became overtly psychotic. He developed delusional beliefs about the therapist and his girl friend. Active interpretation of his rage, self-destructiveness, and primitive defenses did not reduce his symptomatology. According to Kernberg's criteria, it is possible that this patient had underlying psychotic structure. Over a long period of time, the patient eventually recompensated.

Here is another example. Mr. Tilden let slip a disparaging remark about the therapist's country of origin. This comment was made in passing, and at least, on the surface, was directed against someone else. The therapist chose to explore the comment because the sessions had recently seemed quite empty and superficial and she believed that it would be useful to explore the patient's aggressive feelings. When Dr. T asked him about his remark, he became hostile. Why was she picking on his comment? Other things were more important to discuss. Why did Dr. T always have to be in charge of what he talked about? Mr. Tilden insisted that Dr. T not interfere with his talking again. When Dr. T pointed out the patient's need to control her behavior, Mr. Tilden became even more angry. He called her corrupt and domineering. He insisted that Dr. T wanted to control him, and that she wanted to pursue her point until he knuckled under. Mr. Tilden's positive feelings about Dr. T seemed to disappear. Dr. T pointed out his tendency to see her as all bad when he was angry, and to assume that she was feeling as hostile to him as he was to her.

At this point, Dr. T stopped talking and listened. The patient continued to bristle, but also sporadically acknowledged that there was a hostile side to him. In the next session, he spontaneously talked about his feelings of hatred and said that it was a very painful subject to get into. He knew that he had destructive feelings, he said, but he didn't like the way the therapist was pointing them out. He realized that he avoided discussing this side of himself, and thought this would be a slow process. If Dr. T kept cornering him about these feelings, he was not going to be able to discuss them. In any event, to talk about these feelings with the therapist would make him very vulnerable. It was scary to be exposed to someone. It was also scary to admit how much he needed from Dr. T and how much he wanted her to soothe him.

Mr. Tilden and his therapist went on to talk about both the patient's angry feelings and his defensive use of cryptic language to distance himself from her.

The cases presented above demonstrate very different therapeutic outcomes. Transference interpretations of primitive defenses and impulses did not seem to help Ms. Chen or Mr. Martin. Both seemed to be in some kind of extremis in which they needed to maintain the view that destructiveness was outside them, not inside them, and that they were victims, not perpetrators. Whether this was so because of an intolerance of guilt, or for some other reason, is not clear. Mr. Tilden, on the other hand, did benefit from interpretations of his use of projective identification and omnipotent control. Although he clearly was not pleased to confront his own aggression, he was able to tolerate the blow to his self-esteem that was involved, and able to maintain a positive tie to the therapist.

One can speculate about what makes it possible for one patient to maintain an affectionate tie to the therapist, while another becomes suspicious, withdrawn, or breaks off the relationship altogether. Clearly, most patients, except perhaps the most severely antisocial or autistically withdrawn, seek human contact. However one conceptualizes this need, whether as a form of inborn object seeking (Fairbairn, 1944), as a wish for the validation and soothing of a selfobject (Kohut, 1971), or as a longing for intersubjectivity and communion (Stern, 1985), human beings find comfort in contact with others. However, in order to negotiate an approach to the other, an individual must be able to tolerate frustration, delay, uncertainty, anger, disappointment, disillusionment, rejection, sadness, humiliation, and, at least to some degree, a sense of impotence. Obviously, many factors contribute to this capacity, but narcissistic vulnerability certainly plays a part. If one's sense of powerlessness is too great, or one's feeling of worthlessness too deep, frustration becomes a mortifying experience. It may feel like a humiliating submission to tolerate the usual slings and arrows of everyday life as one tries to make contact with others. Such frustrations and deprivations cease to have accidental meaning, but rather are seen as specific commentaries on the worthlessness of the self, which is the patient's view to begin with.

Both Ms. Chen's and Mr. Martin's paranoid episodes began with blows to their self-esteem. Ms. Chen spoke of her "fractured image," and how, years before, she had felt that her mind was literally composed of shit. Paranoid reactions to feelings of worthlessness solve several psychic dilemmas. First, they locate the badness in another person, by means of denial and projection. "They" are worthless, cruel, guilty, or evil. Second, they establish a distance between the self and the object which protects against further "impingements" (Winnicott, 1960b) from the outside. The less one values the other, and the less contact one has, the less that other can hurt and shatter one's fragile sense of ongoing being.

A chronic paranoid stance may represent a compromise between irresistible wishes for contact, soothing, comfort, and communion and inescapable fear of humiliation, worthlessness, and agonizing impingement. While the individual experiences the other as hostile and threatening, and maintains a guarded distance, still there is some ongoing relationship, if only in fantasy. Excessive closeness and therefore vulnerability is avoided, while the experience of human importance is maintained (Auchincloss and Weiss, 1992).

In contrast to Ms. Chen and Mr. Martin, Mr. Tilden was able to respond to interpretation. Although he felt frightened, embarrassed, guilty, and vulnerable, still he persisted in trying to establish a basis for soothing, nurturing contact. Precisely why he and not the others were able to do this is not clear. One can speculate that he experienced some basic nurturing in his development that sustained the hope of benign contact. One can speculate about inborn or developmentally acquired differences in

destructiveness, or the way in which destructiveness is metabo-
lized psychically. One can imagine that the capacity for *self* soothing and turning to the self for love and comfort varies among
children as they grow, and that such self-soothing permits hope
for contact to survive in secret. There are so many factors that
influence the capacity to preserve faith in loving and being loved
in human relationships that it is difficult to pinpoint which of
these factors operate in a specific case. What I have said about
the vulnerability to paranoid withdrawal and the loss of faith in
human goodness, really is descriptive. What in development fos-
ters or kills the capacity for such faith remains mysterious.

Chapter 6

Theory

In this chapter, I will present some theoretical ideas about symbol and concept use in schizophrenia, the disturbance of the sense of boundary in these patients, and the dynamics of paranoia. What I will discuss concerns psychological mechanisms and defensive processes. I will present some thoughts about how psychological factors affect such schizophrenic psychopathology as concreteness of thought, hallucinations, delusions, disturbances of boundary, paranoia, and looseness of association. Before this can be done, we must consider a plausible theory of the interaction between thought, perception, affect, and language in normal individuals.

THE RELATIONS BETWEEN PERCEPTION, AFFECT, THOUGHT, AND LANGUAGE IN NORMAL PSYCHOLOGY

Disturbances of symbol use and concept formation in schizophrenia have been discussed by numerous authors from varying theoretical perspectives. Some writers have focused on the equating of the symbol and the object symbolized (Klein, 1930; Angyal, 1944; Little, 1957; Searles, 1965). Other writers have also referred to the way such dysfunctional symbol use results in "concreteness" of thought (Little, 1957; Arieti, 1974; Searles, 1979). Disturbed symbol and concept use have profound effects on the patient's capacity to perceive, comprehend, represent, imagine, and communicate experience. Schizophrenic patients may live in a world of bizarre and private internal sensations and imagery. They may feel bewildered about the meaning of the social world

151

around them, and may feel affectively isolated because of these disturbances.

Several writers have described the way in which thought in schizophrenics appears to be either permeated by or at times replaced by body states or sensations (Freud, 1915; Searles, 1979). Searles called this *desymbolization*. In referring to a patient who, instead of thinking, experienced sensations, he wrote, "She evidently experienced it not as a figurative thought concept, but concretely as a somatic sensation" (1965, p. 582). Searles gives another example of a woman who felt jealous in the context of a romantic triangle between herself, the female hospital staff, and the doctors. Instead of experiencing the *cognition* that she was involved in a romantic triad, she *perceived* the pupils of her doctor's eyes as being triangular (Searles, 1979, p. 17).

I have provided a number of similar examples in chapter 4. When Ms. Chen felt that the therapist was having too much influence over her, she said that she felt that a dental instrument was poking at her skull. She believed that her therapist did not value her and that her self-esteem had been injured. Instead of realizing that her self-image had been affected, she *perceived* that her body had been altered. Ms. Bender concluded that Dr. M was annoying her with his persistent questions. Instead of conceptualizing this as such, she "saw" a piece of abrasive sandpaper behind Dr. M's head.

In these cases, the patient's images, fantasies, and thoughts somehow become transformed into somatic perceptions—they become *perceptualized*. This perceptualization has enormous consequences. The patient's experience of conceptual and emotional life becomes collapsed, flattened, and compressed. Feelings and thoughts with all their meanings, depth, and resonances become concretized into sensations and perceptions which were not designed to contain them. These sensations thus become "uncanny" or "bizarre" in that they are not only exaggerated versions of sensory processes but, beyond that, contain "surplus meaning" (Ricoeur, 1976). Bion (1957) refers to them as "bizarre objects." Searles wrote that the patient's "perceptual experience is grossly distorted" (1965, p. 581).

Certainly one consequence of the perceptualization of thought is a compromise of reality testing. Obviously, if the patient is under the sway of bizarre and uncanny experiences, he becomes preoccupied and inattentive to the usual perceptual cues. Perception cannot be reliably used to signal *external* stimulation alone. The boundary between internal and external sources of stimuli is thus confused. Moreover, since concept formation (which to a large extent depends upon a social and consensual building up of word meanings [Vygotsky, 1934; Stern, 1985]) is disturbed, the patient's link to conventional social meaning is disrupted. Accordingly, his capacity to evaluate the social criteria of reality is compromised.

This process is analogous to dream formation described by Freud (1900, chapter 7). The dream process attempts to render the complex symbols of preconscious and conscious thought into *visual* images. These ideographs are then experienced perceptually. In schizophrenia, conceptual meaning is rendered not only visually, but, apparently, by audition, touch, smell, taste, pressure, and internal sensory experiences.

Schizophrenic thought is not only perceptualized or sensationalized,[1] it is rendered concrete, and patients have difficulty imagining people, objects, or experiences which are not in the here-and-now (Goldstein, 1944). In these patients, there seems to be a disturbance of the inner world of representation, distinct from perception, in which memory, wish, fantasy, and image can develop and interact. Goldstein (1944) observed, "[There is] an absence of generic words which signify categories or classes" (p. 25).

How can the process of perceptualization be understood? The answer may lie in the path along which perception, image, and thought are developed. This leads us to consider the observations of Spitz, Piaget, and Vygotsky.

For Piaget and Inhelder (1969) and Spitz (1965), the first few weeks, if not months, of life are characterized by an inchoate sensory display of images and sensations which swirl around the infant. Piaget and Inhelder (1969, p. 70) refer to this as a "tableux of reabsorbed objects."[2] At some point (within weeks or months,

---

[1]In this discussion, "perceptualizing" refers to a process by which sensory receptors oriented toward the *external* world (usually distance receptors) generate images. Spitz (1965) terms these sensations "diacritic." "Sensationalizing" refers to the generating of images associated with *internal* somatic impressions, such as hunger or proprioception. Spitz calls these "coenesthetic" sensations.

[2]Spitz (1965, p. 56) compares the experience of formerly blind patients after cataract surgery to what he infers to be the infant's experience early on. At first, such newly sighted

depending on the sense involved) out of this inchoate experience, certain perceptions coalesce. They stand out from their surroundings[3] and become the focus of attention. In terms of sight, the infant is able to identify the boundaries or borders of the visual object, distinguish it from surrounding phenomena, and attend to it. Before this, says Spitz (1965, p. 59), "the *apperceptive* function is not yet available." He adds, "In this sense, the newborn does not perceive; in this sense perception proper is predicated upon apperception" (p. 43). He continues, "Perception, in the sense in which adults perceive, is not present from the beginning; it must be acquired, it must be learned" (p. 56). Goldstein (1944) also refers to the process of figure–ground discrimination in his discussion of schizophrenic thought.

The capacity for apperception, whether developed over time (Spitz, 1965; Piaget and Inhelder, 1969) or immediately available, is the basis for one of the child's first acts of communication: pointing (Stern, 1985). In the act of pointing, the child designates a "syndrome" of perceptions which characterize a delimited object, and refers it to the parents' attention. Later the use of words (at first proper names, and still later on, class names) take over the function of the motor act of pointing.

Now, in the infant, according to Spitz, there are two systems of perception. He refers to one as the coenesthetic system, and to the other as the diacritic system. Coenesthetic experience has to do primarily with internal sensations from the viscera or proprioceptive organs. These sensations tend to be diffuse, unbounded, and unlocalized. Diacritic sensations, by contrast, come from the periphery, and are more circumscribed and focal; they are *intensive* rather than *extensive*. After the development of apperception, the infant possesses the capacity to form a perceptual or sensory image. These images may be visual, acoustic, or tactile. While they may be associated with, or arise in connection with, internal or external sensation, they are not themselves sensations, but are mental contents—either registrations of those sensations, or reproductions of those registrations.[4]

---

patients saw vague and blurry visual forms, but could not distinguish shapes, much less recognize objects. He quotes a report about one such patient: "She saw but it did not mean anything. She was not even positive that these new sensations were coming through her eyes." According to one patient, "everything appeared dull, confused and in motion."

[3]Vygotsky (1934) calls this "bracketing."

[4]For Piaget (Piaget and Inhelder, 1969), all such images are the result of an *active* sensorimotor process. Stern (1985) holds that such experiences are registered and form

With the development of the mental image (often at first, a visual one), mental life takes on a new character. For Piaget (Piaget and Inhelder, 1969), visual images occur at about the same time as the use of verbal symbols, that is, at about 18 months. Both visual image and verbal symbol can evoke the picture of a phenomenon which is not immediately present in time or space. Possibilities for conceptual thought, imagination, anticipation, memory, and mental operations in general expand enormously. This is the time when reproductive memory first appears. For Piaget, reproductive memory is distinct from the earlier sensorimotor scheme. Before reproductive memory, the sensorimotor scheme is, in effect, its own memory. For Stern, the distinction between recognition memory and reproductive memory is not so clear-cut. Some form of reproductive memory—"cued" memories—may occur very early on, considerably before 18 months. In Stern's account, however, such memories do not seem to be the product of sensorimotor action so much as in Piaget's formulation. As a result, they are not subject so much to distortion based on wishes or other factors. In any case, the child can now use a self-generated mental signal (an image), to stand for the perception of external objects and their relations as well as such internal phenomena as affect states, thinking, and memory. The child becomes capable of imagination, fantasy, anticipatory thought, and certain mental operations (Piaget and Inhelder, 1969). The child can now portray to himself events and objects which are not present in space and time. His mental representations may include images of the past or future, affect states and fantasies rather than external perceptions, or somatic sensations alone.

This image-forming function is extremely important and complex. For Piaget, it consists of an "internalized imitation" (Piaget and Inhelder, 1969). Within its own mental environment, the child actively reproduces certain perceptual or sensory experiences which once arose from actual external or internal physical events. Piaget says, "The image which occurs in the image-memory constitutes an *internalized imitation* (1969, p. 83, emphasis

---

the basis of recognition memory. These memories are not necessarily the result of an active process, and thus, one cannot speak of the infant fantasizing at this point. Accordingly, one cannot speak of the infant being capable of fantasy distortion. Stern argues from this, that the infant's perception of his environment is essentially a realistic one, and that distortions of it enter at a much later, verbal stage.

added). He adds that the image "may even elicit *sensations* in the same way as an imagined movement elicits muscular contractions" (p. 69).

To put this in other words, the child creates sensory experiences in the form of images which he uses as symbols for thought. The capacity for sensation, which begins with a strong receptive component[5] (with due respect for the active aspects of apperception and sensorimotor perception) now is pressed into service more actively, to generate sensory stimuli to be used as symbols. These sensory stimuli become the "media" of thinking, separate from thought content. Thinking can occur in a visual medium (i.e., as visual thought or dreams), an acoustic medium (i.e., words or verbal thinking), and perhaps other media as well. Each individual, in effect, is an "artist," who creates a plastic inner world out of visual, acoustic, and other perceptions and sensations, adapted for the purpose of thinking.[6]

One may wonder if those visual images which begin with external perception in some way are "transitional phenomena" (Winnicott, 1953). While they begin in some sense as "given" by the outside world, they are also taken over by the child in his imaginative play. This realm of "mental space" may be a "transitional space" in which the child exercises control over these sensory images. In fact, one may consider that the boundary between external and internal worlds consists not only of the skin and oral mucosa, but also in the "space" between the sensory consequences of the object on the perceptual system and the active reproduction of these experiences. In any case, it is tempting to think of the mind as a transitional space in which the child omnipotently plays with images of reality in accordance with his own needs and wishes. In schizophrenic patients with concreteness of thinking and poverty of ideas, this omnipotent play may be disturbed and the existence of this independent dimension of commentary upon reality is lost. The capacity of the child, and later the adult, to recruit sensory experience in the service of

---

[5]Once again, there is a difference between Piaget's account and Stern's.

[6]Stern (1985) has written about "amodal perception," a memory storage mechanism and even representation mechanism which is independent of particular sensory modalities. There need be nothing contradictory about the existence of both modal and amodal forms of representation. For our purposes, however, we are trying to understand how the schizophrenic patient *perceptualizes* his thought processes, and for this we must trace out a link to the *perceptual* components of thought.

thinking will have a bearing on the subject of the schizophrenic's perception of thought. In order to perceptualize, the patient must have a "perceptualizing apparatus," that is, a mechanism that can convert mental contents into sensory images. In the image forming process described by Piaget we can find such a mechanism. This notion is supported by a good deal of recent neuroscientific evidence. Evidence from studies of brain damaged patients, and from PET scan studies of mental imagery suggest that when an individual tries to evoke a mental image of a past event, or an event in fantasy, he generates images in the perceptual nervous system (Farah, 1988, 1989; Kosslyn, 1988; Kosslyn, Alpert, Thompson, Maljkovic, Weise, Chabris, Hamilton, Rauch, and Buonanno, 1993). Other work has demonstrated that actively generated motor and perceptual sensory elements are also implicated in schizophrenic auditory hallucinations (McGuire, Shah, and Murray, 1993; Waddington, 1993).

If we are to understand, however, how the enormous complexity of abstract thinking can be compressed into concrete sensation, we must understand something about how thought evolves from concrete image to abstract concept. The work of Vygotsky provides some guideposts.

Vygotsky (1934) described the visual organization of concept formation. He described the progression of thinking in categories from "congeries" to concepts. At first, the child groups together anything in its visual field. The elements have a subjectively experienced relation, but this is determined only by their chance congregation in the child's visual field. Later, the child organizes his visual percepts in ways that have more to do with their inherent characteristics. Early on objects may be classified on the basis of associative links (sensory links based on size, shape, or color, etc.) or they may be grouped in "collections" based on their practical relationships (e.g., baseball, bat, and glove). Vygotsky described other forms of linkage between objects (e.g., "chain complexes," "diffuse complexes," and complexes based on "pseudoconcepts"), but the essential point is that the links are not made on the basis of abstract class concepts.[7]

---

[7]Red objects may be classed together on the basis of the red appearance of each, but the child does not have an abstract category for the *concept* "redness" apart from specific and concrete red objects that he sees.

Finally, the child arrives at a linking principle which abstracts a quality from specific objects and generates a *class concept*. The class concept is not simply a proper name for the object, that is, a sound which is taken as an acoustic property of the object itself before there is a representational world. A concept is an abstracted form (Langer, 1967) which defines a class to which elements may belong. Members of a class share some similar form (e.g., grandfather clocks, metronomes, and swings are members of the class "oscillating objects"). The appreciation of "form" and the mental connecting of similar forms or patterns is the basis of class concept formation and abstract thought, whether verbal or logicomathematical. Langer writes, "some kind of knowledge of logical forms . . . is involved in all understanding of discourse . . ." (1967, p. 32). She continues, "The power of recognizing similar forms, i.e., the power of discovering analogies *is* logical intuition" (p. 33).

Now, as the child develops class concepts, he is also developing his use of verbal symbols (according to Piaget [Piaget and Inhelder, 1969] conceptual thought is not identical with verbal representation). Language is an enormous source of images and symbols which can be used for concept formation and communication. It accelerates the child's building up of a representational world. Many authors have noted (Piaget and Inhelder, 1969; Stern, 1985) the way in which language is built up by interactions between parent and child. The child is taught about a social world of agreed upon conventional meanings. A cat is called a "cat," not a "tree." Moreover, those experiences which are public, observable, and easily attached to words gain privileged access to the lexicon. Subjective states, especially the details of private and idiosyncratic experiences, tend to be assigned fewer words and concepts. Says Goldstein (1944), "Language in general in our civilization is more stereotyped and not rich in words to express the specificity of concrete situations" (p. 29).

Thus, in learning verbal symbols, the child gains something and loses something. He gains access to the world of class concepts, to a world of social and historical meanings, and to a verbally mediated picture of the internal states of others. However, he may lose focus on his "unsocialized" capacity to experience the world in an immediate and fresh way, one true to his unique and idiosyncratic self. Langer refers to socialized conceptual knowledge as *knowledge about* in contrast with unique and immediate *knowledge of* (Langer, 1967, p. 22). She uses the term *concept* to refer to socially learned abstract symbols, and *conception* to refer to an individual's private (and not necessarily verbal) way of seeing things (pp. 65–66). This distinction will be important later when I discuss a formulation concerning delusions.

Before turning attention once again to symptomatology in schizophrenic adults, it is necessary to say a word about affects. Obviously, the subject of affect theory is vast and very complicated. It could easily be the subject of many volumes in itself. Here, I simply want to note the important relationship between affects and cognitions. A variety of primary affects, present at birth, have been identified. Among them are happiness, sadness, fear, anger, disgust, surprise, interest, and shame. At first these states have little to do with the infant's cognition or his awareness of *meaning*. Rather, they are biologically rooted capacities for responding to internal and external signals. They have discharge and communicative (i.e., signal) significance and have a variety of adaptive functions. It is only later that affects become connected with cognitions. At this later stage, affects are elicited not only by physical or behavioral phenomena such as hunger or touch, but by cognitions and their associated meanings as well. When the child sees the door open and a nonfamiliar arm begin to enter, he develops a cognition about the arrival of a baby-sitter, and this means that a separation from his mother is imminent. (This process is not one simply of conditioning. Novel stimuli can evoke affective responses depending on the meanings with which they are associated.)

Moreover, affects themselves are structured by cognitions. The affects we are used to dealing with in psychotherapy and psychoanalysis seem to be complex combinations of physiologic responses and cognitions. Envy, contempt, jealousy, pity, and gratitude, for example, all come about because the individual concludes something about the interpersonal world which confers a meaning. If I am envious, for example, I must have a concept of an "other" who possesses objects or qualities which I do not have, but which I value. This is not equivalent in its structure to a "fight–flight" response which is more instinctive, constitutionally programmed, and not necessarily mediated by cognition and meaning. These more complicated affect states (e.g., envy and jealousy) can be understood as existential "stances" or "positions" taken by the individual in the face of an environment which has meaning. They are unlike earlier affect states that consist more simply of biologically inherited potentials for discharge and signaling that can be triggered by social releasers.

After this brief detour through image and concept formation, language acquisition, and affect development, I would like to return to the adult schizophrenic and his symptoms.

DECONCEPTUALIZATION AND ITS RELATION TO CONCRETENESS OF THOUGHT AND HALLUCINATION

Much has been written about disturbances in the patient's affective life. Sometimes affects appear precipitously and seemingly outside the patient's control, or, usually in more chronic patients, affects appear blunted (Bleuler, 1911) or absent altogether. Affects are very disturbing to many schizophrenic patients, whether their own or others, and many authors have commented on the techniques patients use to defend themselves against emotion. Many writers have held that schizophrenic symptomatology, at least in part, serves as a defense against intolerable affects (Eissler, 1953b, 1954; Will, 1975; Searles, 1979, p. 16).

One way in which a patient can protect himself against painful emotion in a social context is to withdraw, and certainly many schizophrenic patients are withdrawn. Another is to blunt or destroy the inner experience of emotion resulting in feelings of inner deadness (Eissler, 1953b, 1954). I would suggest that there is another method of defense which has far more extensive consequences than social withdrawal or emotional flattening. I will call this defense *deconceptualization* (I will use the term *deconceptualization* and *desymbolization* interchangeably unless otherwise specified).[8]

---

[8]It is evident that most human thinking tends most to lean on or recruit visual and acoustic images for its functioning. We preferentially use visual and acoustic images to stand for names and class concepts. Is there a reason why this should be so? Why, for example, should we not "think" in tactile, proprioceptive, olfactory, or taste images? Spitz's formulation concerning diacritic and coenesthetic sensation suggests an answer. Diacritic sensations tend to be more precise and focal, and may be better suited to "stand for" or symbolize specific objects or ideas in thought. Effective social communication depends upon precise and delimited concepts, and it may be that the fact that diacritic sensations (e.g. visual images, acoustic images) are focal makes them more serviceable to represent specific ideas. Moreover, diacritic images arise from *distance* receptors rather

For schizophrenics, affects, including painful ones, are stirred up by cognitions which include abstract class concepts. These cognitions and their attendant meanings evoke powerful associations based upon both unconscious laws of association and conscious, conceptual relations. The resonances and overtones of concepts add intensity and breadth to our thought, and have powerful affective consequences. We experience emotion, not only because of events that physically impinge on our bodies, but because of events that may be far away or even imaginary but which have conceptual meaning for us. The entire realm of fantasy and its consequence for our affective experience depends on the fullness and intactness of conceptual experience.

Bion (1957) has suggested that because schizophrenics are subject to much emotional pain at the hands of external reality (that is, mainly, social interactions), that they attack the apparatus of awareness. He wrote that the schizophrenic "hates reality and all internal mechanisms that make him aware of it" (1956, p. 35). According to Bion, the schizophrenic attacks his own process of forming conceptual links. It is not that individual thoughts are repressed, but that the mechanism of thinking itself is attacked and dismantled. This dismantling renders schizophrenic thought inchoate.

We can understand this "attack on linking" more specifically as a dismantling of the concept-forming capacity. In a sense, the process of concept formation that Vygotsky (1934) described may be reversed. Thought may be progressively shed of class concepts or even specific proper names and is pushed *backwards into perception and sensation*. Although these perceptions are predominantly acoustic, or visual, they may also at times be tactile, olfactory, or gustatory. The inner realm of thought, the "representational

---

than *proximal* receptors and this may have adaptive consequences for the testing of reality. Generally, sensations arising from the body are more urgent than those arising externally. These are the sensations which signal imperative and preemptive biological need. They not only are more likely to disrupt cognitive functioning than visual or acoustic signals, but it is in the interest of biological adaptation that they not be confused with autogenerated sensations used for thinking. Certainly, if visual and acoustic signals used for thought are confused with perception, an individual's functioning is impaired, and his reality testing compromised. But, in terms of the development of the species, it may be better to confuse thought with visual and acoustic percepts, than with percepts relating to hunger, breathing, sexual satiation, or elimination. It may be for these reasons that, in evolutionary terms, we do not think with our gastric or tactile sensations, but rather with our visual and acoustic ones. To put it another way, we do not think with our stomach and skin; we think with our eyes and ears.

world," is shrunken, flattened, and robbed of color. In Vygotsky's terms, class concepts are replaced by "complex" thinking, based upon perceptual similarities or functional relations. These principles of organization of thought may give way to even earlier "congerie" thinking, in which there is practically no thought at all, but merely visual apperceptions devoid of an organizing principle. Beyond that lies only jumbled sensory experience.

Do schizophrenic patients really experience these phenomena? I have given examples of the perceptualization of experience in earlier chapters. Ms. Bender reported: "It is tough to get a hold of an idea, and bring it to my lips." Ms. Weiss said, "My ability to find words to describe what I feel is gone." Ms. Chen stated that she felt that her therapist had injured her self-esteem (i.e., self-image) and that this had *changed the shape of her body*. On another occasion, Ms. Chen said that her uncle told her not to let men "take you to the cleaners." Her boyfriend had recently helped with her laundry, and she asked if that was okay, given her uncle's warning. It seems that the class concept related to being "taken to the cleaners" had been lost.

I think examples such as these provide evidence of the loss of verbal symbols, the concreteness of thought, and of the substitution of perceptions for thoughts in schizophrenic patients. Is there evidence that these processes are set in motion as a defense against painful affect? Ms. Williams reported that for her being homesick was "not an actual wound, it's worse than that. It's a wound in my feelings." Mr. DeVito said, "It would be better to have a void than feelings sometimes.'

Not only do patients often report that affect is intolerable, but also that, somehow, their cognitive dysfunctions are related to such painful feelings. Over a number of sessions, Ms. Weiss told Dr. E of intense and murderous feelings directed toward Dr. E and others. The intensity and vehemence of this hostility was frightening. After having "come alive" over several sessions, as she discussed her homicidal wishes, her demeanor suddenly changed. Once again, she became torpid and listless, and almost appeared sedated. She reported that she felt her mind had calcified and said, "My mind doesn't work well enough for me to get mad." Dr. E was persuaded that the patient's earlier hostile state was very frightening to her, and it appeared to Dr. E that the patient had "dismantled" her thinking in order to avoid this painful affect. Somewhat later, this same patient stated that there was really nothing any more in her head, just a "fog."

Do patients' bizarre or uncanny perceptions and sensations really contain surplus meanings left over from conceptual thinking? In chapters 4 and 5 I have given a number of illustrations of perceptions which, when explored, seem to yield up affective meanings. The example of the visualized "sandpaper" given earlier in this chapter is prototypic. On some level that was not conceptualized, Ms. Bender felt that the therapist was annoying. This belief was not experienced consciously. It seemed that instead, she *perceived* a piece of sandpaper next to Dr. M's chair. Had Dr. M not inquired, her belief that he was annoying might have been lost to awareness. When therapist and patient explored the details of her sensations, and actively applied word concepts to it, there unfolded affect-laden words such as "abrasive," "irritating," and "pushy." Finally the image of an annoying person appeared and Dr. M could link this with the patient's experience of him.

This formulation of desymbolization, deconceptualization, and perceptualization is important because it provides a rationale for treatment technique. It suggests that we examine the patient's behavior, speech, sensations, and perceptions in detail. Even if speech is idiosyncratic, or the perceptions not consonant with the socially accepted version of reality, we assume that the patient's words may contain bits of fragmented conceptual thought. Our effort is to help the patient focus upon these phenomena, and describe them in as much detail as he is able. In the process, we call upon the patient to use skills of attention, focus, image formations, naming, and concept formation in order to explore these uncanny experiences. These skills may have, for defensive reasons, fallen into disuse. Or, for reasons other than defense,[9] they may have become inaccessible to the patient. In either case,

---

[9]Certainly, it may be the case that there are neuroanatomic and neurophysiologic lesions that underlie the "slippage" from concept use to perception. But even if genetic, anatomic, and neurophysiologic factors are implicated in this process, they may not generate these phenomena directly. They may act anywhere along the anatomic–physiologic–affective–cognitive network. Some individuals may be predisposed to such "slippage" from concept to percept, but actualize this potential only under conditions of severe stress. Some individuals may have a predisposition for attaching the "feeling of reality" (Frosch, 1964) to their perceptualizations, resulting in frank hallucinations rather than the seeing of an image in the "mind's eye." The relationship between biological and psychological factors in these processes is of compelling interest, but, obviously, extremely complex and not well understood.

via techniques such as naming, enlargement, and disclosure of the countertransference, the patient and therapist may be able to refind lost affects and meanings. This process can help the patient, if he is so motivated, to take a step back toward the world of socially shared conceptual meaning.[10]

DISTURBANCES IN THE SELF–OBJECT BOUNDARY

Since the beginning of psychoanalysis, many theorists have held that, at the earliest stages of life, the experience of boundary between self and others is undifferentiated (Freud, 1930; Fairbairn, 1941; Fenichel, 1945; Weissman, 1958; Jacobson, 1964; Spitz, 1965; Mahler, 1968; Schafer, 1968; Piaget and Inhelder, 1969; Kohut, 1971; Kernberg, 1975, Loewald, 1980). In their attempts to understand schizophrenic experience, many writers have referred to disturbances in discriminating between self and other, and inside and outside (Freud, 1911; Fairbairn, 1941; Fenichel, 1945; Jacobson, 1954; Winnicott, 1960b, 1962; Searles, 1965, 1979; Mahler, 1968; Kernberg, 1975).

Authors have differed in their understanding of how the disturbance of boundary comes about. Many understand it to be a regression to an earlier state of undifferentiation (Jacobson, 1964; Mahler, 1968; Searles, 1965, 1979). This may occur because of a breakdown of autonomous functions of the ego (Hartmann, 1953) which leads to a collapse of reality testing and a dedifferentiation which is experienced passively. Or, it may come about as a result of active defenses involving fantasies of fusion and merger of self and object representations (Jacobson, 1964; Mahler, 1968; Kernberg, 1975).

Stern (1985) has suggested that there is no early developmental state of merger or fusion, but from its earliest days, the infant has a rudimentary sense of itself as distinct from others.

---

[10]Clearly, these integrative activities require motivation, and the patient, even if capable, may not want to reexperience affects and meanings which are painful. This process must be accompanied by a focus upon the patient's dynamic reasons for remaining isolated and out of touch. It is difficult to discuss the patient's emotions without a reliable language, however, and it is in order to develop a shared conceptual language that naming, enlargement, and disclosure are used. These techniques are designed to help the patient make a connection with the social, conceptual world.

Stern believes that experiences of fusion, when they occur, arise only after the achievement of a capacity for active fantasy.

Whether they first originate in earliest development, or in later fantasy productions, the sense of a confused demarcation between self and other is prominent in the symptoms of schizophrenic patients. A 50-year-old man came to the clinic one day without an appointment. He wanted to see his therapist, Dr. O, and was clearly upset. I asked him why he had come. He replied, "You know why I'm here, Dr. O; don't play games with me." Dr. O told him that, in fact, he did not know, and could not figure out what the patient was thinking without his telling him. He answered, "Then how did I know to come here today? I knew you wanted me to come. Why else would I come all the way from downtown, when I had better things to do?" Clearly, for this man, the boundary between his thoughts and Dr. O's thoughts was confused.

Ms. Chen often felt that her therapist had entered too far into what she called her "personal space." When this happened, she said, she felt (she had a near sensory perception) that her therapist was pinching her ear with tweezers. Apart from her perceptualizing the concept of intrusion, and apart from its oral connotations, this sensation demonstrates Ms. Chen's fragile sense of coherence in space. She did not have an inner mechanism to somehow establish an effective barrier against the experience of invasion. It is this function, which involves both identifying inner states as belonging to the self, and outer influences as remaining external, which I have referred to earlier as the sense of boundary.

What is the mechanism by which this sense of boundary may become disturbed in psychotic patients? Biological factors could play a role, and defects in a neurophysiologic "stimulus barrier" could affect a sense of what is internal and what is external. As noted above, investigators have theorized about defects in ego functioning (i.e., "regressive dedifferentiation") and active defense springing from conflict. Other somatic factors might also come into play. What I would like to focus on here, however, is another psychological mechanism which may play an important role.

As I suggested in chapter 5, the experience of an intact boundary may be partly rooted in interpersonal affective experience. If an individual finds that his own emotions or thoughts are powerfully influenced by the behavior of another, one may speak of an impaired boundary. For example, if a child's feeling of tranquility is utterly disrupted by his mother's irritable mood, one may say that the child's inner world has been intruded upon by the adult. Some degree of this, obviously, is part of everyday life. But if it occurs with excessive force or frequency, the child may feel that there is no effective brake on the mother's capacity to influence his inner state. He may experience this vulnerability as an absence of boundary.

Stern's work (1985) may provide some help in understanding this mechanism. Stern describes the experience of interaffectivity after the child has developed an intersubjective self. During this period, the child has a powerful need to "know and be known," and deliberately seeks the sharing of experience with an other. Via behaviors which include gestures and vocalizations, the child and his mother send signals to each other. If these signals are reasonably well matched in form, intensity, and other characteristics, a sense of "interpersonal communion" develops in which the child feels that his mother has, in some way, "understood" his subjective experience. Stern believes that the mother must match the formal qualities of her child's experience, what he terms the "vitality affects," in order to signal a matching. *Attunements* is the term Stern uses for the mother's responses which mirror the form and intensity of her child's inner experience.

Now, if the mother is motivated and able to perform attunements which approximate her child's inner state, the child experiences a "going on being." If, however, the mother's gestures do not match the child's vitality affects, a "misattunement" occurs, and the child's ongoing subjective experience is interrupted. This interruption may be felt to be very painful by the child. Instead of a satisfying "going on being," the child feels that both the flow of its own functioning, and its communion with the mother have been interrupted. Instead of feeling understood, he may feel very alone. Or he may experience the mother's mismatching as a coercive attempt to control or change his inner state. If such misattunement persists, the child learns that intersubjectivity may lead, not to pleasurable sharing, but to a painful loss of inner peace and continuity.

Interestingly, if misattunements are too far off the mark, they have less impact on the child. In effect, the child may brush them aside and ignore them as being unrelated to himself. If, however, a misattunement appears at first to match the child's vitality affects, it can "gain entry" into the child's experience, only, finally, to disrupt the child's sense of well-being. As noted above, the child may experience the faulty attunement as coercive and controlling. He may feel that the parent does not want him to feel his own feelings. He may not only feel alone, but under the pressure of his need to reestablish an interpersonal communion, he may try to comply with the pressure he perceives. Thus, he may tone down his joy, he may feign happiness when sad, he may pretend pleasure when there is none. In effect, he may develop a "false self" (Winnicott, 1960a). His actual subjective experience, his "true self," may be driven underground and become secret. Stern (1985) points out that the "not-me" of Sullivan (1964) may correspond to these disavowed subjective states. It should be noted that, according to Stern, if the mother matches the child's inner state too completely, or too frequently, the child may experience a kind of psychic transparency, in which he believes that his thoughts and feelings are immediately accessible to the parent. In this case, there is no privacy.

It is very tempting to connect Stern's discussion of the child's intersubjective experience with Klein's notion of projective identification (Klein, 1946). For Klein, the individual who uses projective identification attempts, in fantasy, to enter the mind of the other, with the wish to control them or destroy them from the inside. Whether this fantasy actually exists in adult patients or not, the child may feel like the victim of such an attempt. According to Stern, the child experiences misattunements as coercive efforts to enter his mind and control his inner experiences. It is not a great speculative leap to imagine that in his effort to adapt, the child may wish to turn passive into active, and begin to entertain fantasies of entering into and controlling the minds of others. This early interpersonal experience may also be the basis for later delusion of control and thought broadcasting (Schnieder, 1959). It may also help us to understand delusions concerning the capacity of others to read one's mind.

This detour through Stern's work, I think, sheds light on our understanding of the sense of boundary. While we may or may not believe that neurophysiological factors affect the discrimination between self and others, or inside and outside, it does appear that early interpersonal experiences can influence the subjective experience of a boundary. The child's experience of "transparency" reflects a concern that there is no *cognitive* barrier between the contents of his mind and other people's perceptions. The sense of coercion related to misattunements may generate a concern that there is no *affective* barrier between his own ongoing feelings states and the affective intrusions of others. Even without the concept of attunement, we know that others can have profound effects upon our moods and feelings. If we cannot somehow mitigate the impact of the effects (if, for example, we cannot help feeling guilty after a parental criticism, or we cannot help feeling envious when a colleague discusses an achievement, etc.), then functionally, there is a reduced sense of boundary.

Do these formulations about the sense of boundary apply in the clinical setting? I think there is evidence that they do.

Mr. Tilden came in from the waiting room. He said that he had a very important dream and had remembered all the details in the morning, but now had forgotten it. He started to talk about something else very briefly, then paused and said that he didn't know what else to say. The therapist asked how he understood his forgetting his dream. The patient became furious. She did this all the time, he said. Did she *want* to injure him? Why was she always trying to force *her* ideas of what they should talk about on him. Did she think the session was there for *her* benefit? He said that the therapist was "toying" with him and "cornering him." He declared that, now, he didn't trust her. He went on like this for perhaps fifteen minutes. Finally, he said, "I can't afford to indulge myself in being so angry with you because I need you on my side."

This patient's rage at the therapist could be understood as a reaction to a feeling of an interruption of his "going on being," and was an "impingement" in Winnicott's terms (1960a). He experienced her as intrusive, self-centered, and even actively malevolent. In referring to her "cornering" him, it seems he was making reference to what Stern calls the "coercive" effect of misattunements. In his view, the therapist's image of him was too narrow for his sense of full subjectivity to be comfortable with, and he would not accept a too restrictive confinement of his self. The patient appeared to feel that his therapist had violated his sense of integrity in some way. Clearly this feeling was consistent with a lifetime of feeling "squelched" by family and friends.

Seemingly, this patient had three options. He could withdraw from interpersonal contact; he had done this many times before, falling into prolonged silences. He could submit and act as if nothing had happened, developing a false "cooperative" demeanor, or he could actively protest. This last option may have been the most growth promoting, and in this instance, was the one he chose.

Another important feature of Mr. Tilden's experience was his sense of need and impotence. He had an unpleasant choice. He could continue to stand by his sense of self and protest, risking a loss of contact or communion with the therapist. Or, he could "disavow" a very meaningful self-experience in order to maintain contact. Often, he experienced this last choice as humiliating. He felt shame over being such a "sucker" and felt that he was "weak."

Mr. Tilden felt the choice between humiliating surrender or defiant aloneness to be either/or, and part of the therapeutic work was to help him understand that the therapist's "misattunements" were not intentional, and that, in any case, he was free to stand by his sense of self and protest when he needed to, and that maintaining a relationship did not mean that he had to abandon his sense of integrity.

Mr. Tilden's belief that he had to adopt a "false," compliant self to maintain contact with his therapist had a variant. On another occasion, he said, he wanted *the therapist* to be nice, so that they could get back to having a good relationship. Why did *he* always have to submit? Instead of denying the meaning of his own self-experience, the patient wanted the therapist's position to change. Instead of a kind of "masochistic merger" based on a false self, he wanted a change to come from the therapist. One might wonder whether this mechanism, at least in part, lies behind what has been termed "omnipotent control" (Kernberg, 1975). The patient desperately wants to maintain positively toned feelings toward the therapist. If he feels a misattunement, he has two choices: he can develop a submissive false self; or try to get the therapist to act in such a way as to not stir up more misattunement. The patient, clearly, will have very specific ideas about how the therapist should behave in order that he, the patient, return to a subjective feeling of attunement.

Klein (1946) and Kernberg (1975) believe that projective identification results from an intrapsychic fantasy. I am suggesting here that projective identification may have an interpersonal origin as well, arising in the context of one person's affective impact on another.

It is important to note that the disturbance of boundary discussed above does not necessarily imply a loss of reality testing. The capacity to discriminate between self and other, or between internal and external sources of perception, or the capacity to appreciate the social criteria of reality (Kernberg, 1975, 1984), are not necessarily frankly impaired when there is a sense-of-boundary disturbance. In its extreme forms, however, the experience of coerced inner states, or of transparency may contribute to intense feelings of interpersonal lack of control and lack of autonomy from emotional influence. These feelings are not, in themselves, psychotic. However, their deconceptualized and perceptualized representation in the form of the experience of a common skin, or thinking the other person's thoughts, or feeling the other person's pain, and so on, does typify the psychotic experience of self-object dedifferentiation. There is a core of interpersonal affective reality in the psychotic experience of the loss of boundary. But this interpersonal experience might not lead to the loss of the self-object distinction which defines psychosis, were it not for the form in which it is represented. This form arises from the process of deconceptualization and perceptualization. It is these processes which result in the concrete, subjectively felt experience of dedifferentiation and merger.

A FORMULATION CONCERNING PARANOIA

What has been said above about the sense of boundary, I think, bears directly on the experience of paranoid patients. The sense of a shattered boundary and the vulnerability of the subjective sense of self, lies at the center of the paranoid patient's experience of himself, and contributes to his feelings of rage. It seems that for some paranoid patients, it is neither easy nor acceptable to develop a false, compliant, social self. Perhaps for such patients, hiding a "true" self away is not enough to protect against a feeling of annihilation. Perhaps the integrity of such a hidden true self is felt to be too precarious and unreliable. Whatever the case may be, such patients react to impingements or intrusions on their integrity with violent rage.[12]

Set against this is the individual's need not only to be a self, but *him* self. This conflict was described by Mr. Tilden, who had a number of paranoid trends. Unable to fall back on a false-self solution, the patient can either withdraw or protest. But if the conflict is more intense, it may take on a more overtly paranoid form. Objects may be experienced as intensely invasive, impinging, dysregulating, and shattering of the individual's sense of cohesion. In this case, the person experiences an urgency about escaping a form of agony (Winnicott, 1962, 1963b). The forms of withdrawal and the forms of protest may be correspondingly intense. Withdrawal may take the form of an abrupt and profound social isolation. Ms. Chen had very little contact with anyone. Her one contact, apart from the relationship with her therapist, was with a boyfriend, with whom she stayed for several months. On one occasion, he made an unwanted remark. The patient reacted with rage. She abruptly and permanently ended the relationship with him, with her employer, and with her therapist. It seemed that her experience of violation and impingement was so intense, that her interpersonal world had to be reduced practically to zero in order that her sense of self feel safe.

Ms. Chen was very suspicious of transference interpretations. She felt that her therapist was being "too personal" and brushed aside clarifications and interpretations. Her therapist understood this not to be evidence of an incapacity for transference, but of a very particular transference disposition. The patient was frightened that the therapist would somehow take control over her. She experienced the meaning of this in perceptualized form as a dental instrument poking at her skull, or copper wires attached to her body.

Ms. Chen's withdrawal stands in contrast to the reciprocal reaction of rageful protest. (Actually her ending her relationships with boyfriend, employer, and therapist expressed both withdrawal and protest.) Ms. Chen often reacted with rage when she

---

[12]For another way of understanding Mr. Tilden's need to control his therapist's behavior, see chapter 5, "Paranoia." I do not think that these two views are necessarily at odds.

felt that her "personal space" had been invaded. Mr. Martin simi-larly, responded with fury when he felt that his therapist didn't understand him, or care about him, or if he felt that his therapist was not on his side.

The response of rage accomplishes several things and may be the preferred one. First, it creates a distance which may bring relief from a sense of impingement. Second, it may help consoli-date a fragile sense of self. Mr. Tilden said, "Not agreeing with you is the only thing that keeps me sane." Third, it can be a response to a sense of powerlessness. Aggression may naturally call up senses of self which involve activity, potency, and control. Finally, an ongoing hostile relation establishes distance, but also maintains (even if distantly, and only in fantasy) some sense of ongoing connection (Auchincloss and Weiss, 1992). The thread of interpersonal communion, even if only in fantasy, and even if attenuated and charged with anger, is still maintained.[13]

Certain particular cognitions may accompany the patient's sense of impingement. Certainly, it would consolidate and ratio-nalize the patient's experience for there to be a personified "im-pinger." If the individual feels that his inner affective state is being robbed or stolen, this would understandably be comple-mented by the notion that there is a robber behind this process. Ms. Chen reacted angrily to the sense that her therapist had been coercive and hurtful. She said, "Do you want me to be unhappy?" The idea that her therapist was motivated to harm her had appeal. It may be that it is difficult for patients, or people in general, to believe that their agony has been caused by accident or by chance. Certainly, Piaget (Piaget and Inhelder, 1969) tells us that the appreciation of chance is a late event in the development of think-ing in the child.

The formulation described above certainly does not rule out the possibility that part of the patient's sense of a hostile other stems from his own projected rage.

---

[13]It may be that for such patients, the connection to the object is not what might be called "discretionary." The loss of the other does not result in sadness, which can be tolerated and absorbed, but, rather, is experienced as intolerable. It may feel similar to losing an arm or leg. This may be because, developmentally, threats of loss occurred at a time when, in fact, the mother *was* indispensable, as a need gratifying object (A. Freud, 1962), for physiologic regulation, or to satisfy an imperative need for interpersonal affecti-vity and intersubjectivity (Stern, 1985). In any event, the presence of the object may not have been perceived as discretionary.

THE LOSS OF MEANING, THE LOSS OF IDENTITY, AND THE LOSS OF CONTACT WITH THE SOCIAL CRITERIA OF REALITY

I would like to comment on that aspect of reality testing which Kernberg (1975) referred to as the "social criteria" of reality. Kernberg identified the capacity to empathize with these social criteria as one of the cornerstones of intact reality testing. It involves the individual's capacity to appreciate the point of view that other observers have about him.

It would seem that this capacity can only arise after the development of language, which provides a consensually developed, public, and therefore "official" set of meanings (Vygotsky, 1934; Langer, 1967; Stern, 1985). Implicit in the syntax and vocabulary of language is a conventional viewpoint about objects and events, including human behavior and experience. According to Vygotsky (1934), the child can only begin to develop an "objective" view about himself after he has understood language and its socially developed meanings. Language serves as a transition between the outer world of defined and delimited cultural meanings, and an idiosyncratic inner, private world of perception, sensation, affect, and image. According to Vygotsky, the child first learns "public" language ("external speech") and only later applies it to his inner states ("inner speech").

When verbal thought is compromised, as it is in schizophrenia, when concepts are transformed into sensations or perceptions, the individual loses contact with the social and cultural point of view. He no longer participates so fully in his thinking with the point of view of the "average expectable member" of the culture. As a result, his world becomes more private and more autistic. His appreciation of the *social* criteria of reality is compromised.

There is a second factor which may contribute to the loss of empathy with the average social viewpoint. Because in psychotic patients the sense of a cohesive self is disturbed, the patient may have little experience of the feeling of a healthy, coherent self. His fears may be so powerful, his sense of vulnerability so urgent, and his need to act defensively so preoccupying, that he may have little understanding of what an "average expectable self" feels like. It may therefore be quite difficult for him to empathize with the experience of the relatively healthy selves who define what behaviors and affects constitute conventional "normality."

Ms. Chen, who was quite isolated and who experienced her sense of self as extremely threatened, frequently seemed to have little or no idea about why people acted as they did. She would continually ask her therapist why colleagues, acquaintances, or family members would behave in a certain way. Questions such as: "What do you think he meant," and "Why did he say that?" were a regular feature of the meetings. It did not seem to be a contradiction to Ms. Chen to also ask her therapist what she should do in many cases. Despite her extreme sensitivity to coercion and invasion of her "personal space," Ms. Chen's bewilderment about how and especially why people functioned in the social world, led her to invite her therapist to be a kind of anthropological guide to an exotic and bewildering social world.

This sense of living in a strange land is portrayed in Kafka's *The Trial*. K seems utterly bewildered about why his accusers have set upon him, and seems out of touch with and uncomprehending of the behavior of those around him. They have profoundly disturbed his sense of "going on being," but he seems not to be able to understand their language, or to put himself in their shoes.

DELUSIONS

An understanding of the collapse of the inner realm of conceptual thought into concrete images, sensations, and perceptions, and the isolation from the world of social meanings that it brings, may help us understand something about the nature of delusions. By definition, delusions are beliefs which contradict the commonly held views of material reality (e.g., the earth is made of cheese) or social (e.g., Elvis Presley is the President). In discussing the loss of empathy with the social criteria of reality, I mentioned that the inner realm of concept and abstract image had collapsed. When this occurs, the multitude of concepts about social and personal issues that the individual has, also collapses as thought becomes concrete, perceptualized, and sensationalized. Having lost verbal concepts and their well-defined social meanings, the individual must fall back on presocial, prelinguistic forms of thought—idiosyncratic personal images. Vygotsky (1934) called this "autistic" or "alogical" thought. In referring to schizophrenic thinking, Kasanin said, "Things have a personal, not a symbolic value" (Kasanin, 1944). In referring to the public, rather than the private function of language, he wrote, "Language in our civilization is more stereotyped, and not rich in words to express the specificity of concrete situations" (p. 29). Kraepelin (1902) noted that schizophrenics express "complicated, morbid ideas for which no words exist."

Suzanne Langer (1967) referred to the distinction between public and private image when she described the difference between concept and conception. The concept has a publicly shared, delimited meaning. The conception, by contrast, is a private image built up out of personal experience which may or may not find expression in public concepts. It corresponds to what Bertrand Russell called "knowledge of," rather than "knowledge about." Our *concept* of 90 degrees Fahrenheit may have to do with a thermometer whose mercury has risen to a certain level. Our *conception* of such heat may have to do with a particular visual image of shadeless sunlight, or air shimmering off a hot pavement, or the singular sensation in our mouths when we are thirsty.

It is certainly true that private conception and public concept interact. Poets, creative writers, and patients among others try to find ways to express their private conceptions in public, verbal terms. On the other hand, we have all had the experience of discovery when a routine public concept that we have heard repeatedly is connected with a private, immediate experience. We experience something like an epiphany, and the concept comes alive.

Now, when the psychotic patient's conceptual world collapses, it may be replaced by his earlier conceptional world. He may experience images and meaning essentially private to himself. When these meanings replace a public concept, the ground may be prepared for a delusion. We all have private conceptions about our experience, many of which are, by definition, unconscious, because they have limited access to words. These are the images which are subject to the unconscious primary process described by Freud in *The Interpretation of Dreams* (1900). These images undergo characteristic transformations which include displacement, condensation, and symbolization. When an individual substitutes his conception for the cultural concept, and when he attaches a *feeling of reality* (Frosch, 1964) to this conception, a delusion has been formed. His conception is not experienced as a subjective point of view, or a personal slant, but as objectively true.

Mr. DeVito believed that a gangster had entered his heart. When actively psychotic, he believed that this gangster would control his behavior and bring destruction on him. Over the course of several years of work, the following memories emerged: shortly after he started to attend school, he began treatment with a brace to correct congenital hip dysplasia. Sometime after, his sister fell ill and much of the family's time and resources were devoted to her. Still later, a family friend told the patient lurid stories about the Sicilian mob. The patient's ongoing experience of his aunt was that of an involved, even loving, but intrusive and smothering presence. For many years, the patient lived with his aunt and uncle, when he was a patient. His aunt cooked his meals, and worked as a secretary to support him. On one level, the patient understood that his aunt was "only" a person, that even if she was overinvolved, she loved the patient in her own way. This was the level of social *concept*. On another level, he had a *conception* of his aunt as an unstoppable invader who made him feel claustrophobic within his own self, whose presence felt so expanded that it threatened his sense of cohesive self. In this conception, the images of the mechanical disruption in his sense of going on being (the brace) and the cohesion of his self, was linked to a later disruption of his feeling of interpersonal communion and affectivity (his feeling displaced by his sister from being the focus of his parents' attention.) which, in turn, was linked to the frightening experience of his uncle's Cosa Nostra stories. These links are nothing unusual. We all have such irrational linkages in our unconscious conceptional thought.

My hypothesis is that what brought these images to the forefront was the breakdown in the availability of conceptual thought, which in itself permits a link to external human objects. These objects, when internalized, permit the soothing of fear, and the dampening of disintegrative anxiety, and the reduction of primitive defenses (Klein, 1946). Abstract thought can thus symbolically help the individual maintain an affective link to the world of humans. With the loss of *conceptual* links, the patient's *conceptional* links impressed themselves more forcefully on him. In the absence of social concepts, the individual's autistic conceptions hold sway. The soothing internal link to the world of humans fades away, and the individual feels that there are no internal good images of humans. Paranoid and schizoid fears of dissolution, disintegration, and a crescendo of unbearable anxiety may begin to swell.

Still, no matter how anxiety generating, these irrational private links would remain "overvalued ideas" were it not that they were connected with a feeling of reality. The origin and function of the feeling of reality is complex, and not something that can be discussed here at great length, but it seems to be vital for the evolution of the species. Clearly, it is adaptive for living organisms to connect a particular feeling tone to external perception, and even internal sensation. External dangers and urgent internal needs must be attended to and not confused with fantasy, illusion, or "hypochondriacal" experience. In humans, the function of the "feeling" of reality is complicated by the existence of a sensory based, representational life which evolves from perceptions and sensations, which are then used for thinking; that is, visual, acoustic, and other images. Human beings must discriminate between images, fantasies, memories, and concepts on the one hand, and perceptions and sensations on the other. Hartmann (1953) refers to this process as "inner reality testing."

The fact that mental contents exist in such a panoply of images arising from such different sources, constitutes a weak point for the feeling of reality. If sensations and perceptions were the only mental content, mistakes in the feeling of reality and the loss of reality testing would not be so much an issue. This may be the case for animals, who have relatively little symbolic mental life, and who can ill afford to lose contact with reality. Since human mental experience goes far beyond sensation and perception, opportunities expand for confusing fantasy, mental image, and perception.

Clearly also, there are psychodynamic reasons for attaching a sense of reality to nonreal phenomena. We are familiar with this in its negative form in the defense of denial, when a bit of external reality is detached from a feeling of reality, and ignored. We treat the person or event as if it did not exist. Similarly, we can treat our own inner experience as if it were not real, and detach it from a feeling of reality (Klein [1935] refers to the "denial of internal reality"; Jacobson [1967] also refers to this phenomenon). Clinically, we understand that denial and disavowal are used defensively to resolve conflict.

Psychotic patients may use the accentuation of a feeling of reality (rather than its diminution) also in a defensive way to reduce conflict. When under stress, Mr. DeVito felt very much alone, very much in need of being taken care of, and very much in need of rescue from coercive, invasive others. He felt vulnerable, helpless, and controlled. One may hypothesize that because of the loss of a conceptual frame of reference, and because he needed to enlist the help of others, the conception of the brace–abandonment–aunt–family friend–Sicilian–mob–gangster which was preformed in his fantasy, became attached to a feeling of reality. In so doing, the patient felt there was good reason to make an urgent appeal for help and intervention.

One may speculate that just as human beings can reproduce visual and acoustic sensations to use for thinking, so they can reproduce the "feeling tone" which usually accompanies external perception or internal sensation. All perception and sensation must have a distinctive impact on the central nervous system which signals their existence, their "isness." This feeling tone or "isness" sensation goes a long way to establish the "real existence" of a phenomenon. The activity of reality testing proper which is a cognitive act, and not a feeling, is only really a corroboration. The result of this reality testing process, like most psychic phenomena, can be ignored, denied, or rationalized as needs warrant.

When the conceptual world of the psychotic becomes concrete, meanings appear to vanish, but as we have seen, they are not obliterated entirely. Sometimes, they may return in a perceptual or sensory medium in the form of bizarre or uncanny perceptions or sensations. Or, they may return in a cognitive medium, albeit in a nonconceptual (i.e., non class concept) fashion, in the form of ideas of reference and delusions. The poverty of meaning which is such a feature of the schizophrenic's inner life, is the obverse of the surplus of meaning which he experiences in ideas of reference and delusions.

The concretizing of thought may play a role in the phenomenon of "psychotic transference" described by Little (1957) and Searles (1963). The patient who experiences such a transference does not distinguish between the therapist and the image of a figure from his past. This may occur because there is no "past" as an ideational, nonsensory mental content to which to refer when the conceptual world becomes concrete. The patient knows that an intense feeling is being experienced in the present. Yet, he does not have a recoverable past to refer this feeling to. He cannot say, for example, "I feel very tense and frightened like I did when my father criticized me. Moreover, I remember that, earlier today, I had a dream about my father yelling at me. I must be carrying this feeling around with me wherever I go, and I can see that my therapist is not the one evoking it in me." Unlike such an individual, the schizophrenic patient only knows that he is in the presence of his therapist, and that he is experiencing this powerful emotion. Ipso facto, the therapist is implicated in this state and is thought to have evoked it. The patient has thus confused past with present, and "symbol" with object. I place the term *symbol* in quotations, because, in fact, the patient is not truly capable of symbolizing at this point.

LOOSENESS OF ASSOCIATION AND OVERABSTRACTION

The clinical phenomenology of looseness of association may be connected with a patient's defensive need to obscure his meaning. Disjointed speech may occur because the patient is more interested in playing with word sounds than in communicating, or may be more interested in *not* being understood than being comprehensible. However, another mechanism may be at work. Mr. Tilden had some thoughts about his brothers the day before. He wanted to discuss them in his session, but wasn't sure it was a good idea. He said, "I'm afraid the idea will become cold and hard like a fossil." Later on, he said even more obscurely, "When I talk about it (the subject of his brothers), I feel like I'm plugging myself up."

On the surface, these utterances might appear to be "looseness of association" or a variant. They might seem to result from a disturbance of the "synthetic function" of the ego (Nunberg,

1931). However, after some inquiry, Mr. Tilden seemed to be verbalizing a private conception, albeit in an imperfectly conceptual and public way. He felt, as many psychotic patients do, that he had been coerced by his parents who did not care to understand his real self. His mother had appeared sympathetic, and the patient had let her into his emotional life, only to find that his mother consistently had her own agenda and needed the patient to fulfill her own needs. By means of her explosive temper, his mother had made him feel "splintered." Unless the patient's behavior conformed with her image of him, he felt, he could be exposed to an intimidating and self-shrinking barrage.

As the therapist and patient discussed these details, Mr. Tilden referred to a "plugged up Steven" and a "secure Steven." The "plugged up Steven" corresponded to his experience of coercion which made him feel humiliated and angry. The "secure Steven" was a compliant, passive, hedonistic, lazy but seemingly content "false self," disconnected from needs for recognition, dignity, authority, and initiative. The patient was finally able to explain that if he were to force himself to talk about the idea he had over the weekend, it would only feel stale and irrelevant; dead "like a fossil." He would be coercing himself and treating himself as his parents had—"plugging" himself up, metaphorically speaking.

The patient was presenting a private conception in his speech, and had not taken pains to translate it into a public concept. In his case, the capacity for conceptual thought was intact, and conventional verbal concepts were available to him. He was able, when asked, rather easily to translate his conceptional images into conventional language.

For psychotic patients whose conceptual process has become concretized or perceptualized, standard, verbal concepts may not be so available. For them, concrete imagery and perceptions keep autistic conceptions enwrapped in their "personal space." Sometimes this may be intentional. Sometimes, however, the process may have taken its own course, and the patient may be unable to escape a kind of private mental incarceration. He had no verbal concepts to unlock his autistic cell.

Curiously, schizophrenic patients are not only excessively concrete in their thinking, but also, at times, seem to be overly abstract. This may be understood in terms of the delinking of words from their underlying referrants (Freud, 1915). Instead of associating words predictably and reliably, with fixed and agreed upon concepts and meanings, schizophrenic patients seem to detach the verbal signifiers from the signified. Words become used in a kind of "acoustic play"; Klang associations, neologisms, and perseveration are examples. A patient remarked, "The effectuation of the assistance of the dynamism is a constituent of private pursuit."

A number of writers have referred not only to the communication function inherent in language, but the obscuring function as well. Kasanin (1944) wrote, "We find that words, sentences, utterances frequently are a mask for something the speaker *does not want to disclose*" (p. 000, emphasis added). Burnham (1955) speaks of the wish for and fear of communication. Stern (1985) makes a similar point.

Ms. Williams spoke incomprehensibly in the community meeting. She ate napkins and entered into long, obscure speeches. Later, she told me that she spoke so bizarrely to cover up the fact that she was scared.

PRIMITIVE SELF-DESTRUCTIVENESS

I have already referred several times to Stern's formulations concerning the intersubjective self. The experience of interpersonal communion can be one of intense and special joy. When attunements fail, however, a great sense of aloneness can develop, or a coercive interruption of "going on being."

We may extend this a bit, and hypothesize that the child may arrive at a somewhat "paranoid" view. He may feel that the mother *wants* to tone down, diminish, control, or even, somehow, annihilate his core sense of self. As always, he faces the choice between aloneness, false-self formation, or protest. A more ominous choice is also available; that is, the choice of "identifying with the aggressor," and in the service of preserving some kind of "communion" with the patient, actively trying to eradicate his own self-experience. Since the sense of a core self consists of a variety of components (e.g., a sense of spatial and temporal coherence, a sense of affective coherence, a sense of perceptual coherence, and a sense of coherence of agency, among others

[Stern, 1985]) the "undoing" of a sense of self may involve any, or all, of these dimensions. What one might call "masochism in the service of communion" in the adult patient may take a variety of forms: self-destructive passivity, self-destructive affective storms, self-destructive drug-induced perceptual chaos, or self-destructive physical injury. If the patient believes that the other desires his annihilation, he may conclude that only the most complete eradication of his sense of his own self will satisfy his intersubjective partner. The patient may fantasize that by eliminating his sense of self he has eliminated the offending element which has blocked communion with his loved one. He may believe, at least in fantasy, that he can return to a time before there was a sense of self, a time when he did not experience, as such, the agony generated by gross misattunement. Clearly, this process may motivate the dissolution of self-object boundaries which contributes to the further development of psychotic structure.

A PERSPECTIVE ON REALITY TESTING

I would like to offer a brief formulation concerning the way in which the concepts developed in this chapter concerning concept formation, deconceptualization, perceptualization, the sense of boundary, and language use may affect the functions of reality testing. I would like to sketch the ways in which deconceptualization and perceptualization undermine the ability of the ego to test reality. I will use Kernberg's (1975) definition of reality testing as a reference point. Kernberg holds that reality testing consists of three essential components: the capacity to discriminate internal from external sources of perception; the capacity to discriminate self from object; and the capacity to empathize with the social criteria of reality. For brevity's sake, I will present my ideas in outline form.

The Discrimination Between Internal and External Sources of Perception

1. Thought is sensationalized and perceptualized.
2. Since perceptions replace concepts, the distinction between perceptions arising externally, and perceptions arising internally is undermined.

3. The "feeling" of reality may be attached to perceptualizations and add to the sense of their being real.
4. The absence of an inner realm of concept makes it more difficult to refer the perceptualizations back to their original *mental* conceptual source since the world of ideas and meanings no longer exists. These perceptualizations appear to have an obvious, tangible, empiric quality to them. There is no other way of accounting for them—other than that they, in fact, come from the external world—since they are no longer experienced as *subjective* mental phenomena.
5. Concepts which are sensationalized rather than perceptualized, become a source of hypochondriacal experience.

Self-object Discrimination

1. The sense of boundary, which is normally flexible and somewhat permeable, becomes disturbed.
2. This disturbance arises because the individual's sense of self is interrupted by the actions of the other.
3. This interruption is experienced as an impingement.
4. This painful experience leads to a sense of vulnerability to the coercive effect of the other.
5. In itself, this disturbance in the sense of boundary does not constitute a blurring of the boundary between self and other.
6. Only when it is represented in deconceptualized or perceptualized form, is it experienced subjectively as a dedifferentiation, or a loss of the sense of boundary.
7. The loss of boundary may be accelerated by a psychodynamic motive. The individual may wish to eradicate his sense of self in order to affect an intersubjective communion with a destructive other (masochism in the service of communion).

The Social Criteria of Reality

1. The psychotic patient has experienced a collapse of his inner, conceptual world.
2. This means a loss of verbal concepts which link him to the broader, common culture.

3. Thereby, he loses contact with social meanings and points of view.
4. As a result, he is not able to view himself objectively as an average expectable social observer would.
5. This disturbance is compounded by the fact that his sense of a coherent self has been disrupted. Because of this, he has lost touch with, or has never known, what an average expectable coherent self would feel like.
6. The individual thus experiences a bewildering world of social ritual which is opaque to his understanding.
7. His appreciation of the social criteria of reality is, thereby, impaired.

Chapter 7

Working Through

Reporting the results of the therapeutic work with the psychotic patients in this sample is problematic for several reasons. The number of patients involved is small. One must be extremely cautious about generalizing findings from such a limited group. Clinical presentations and responses to interventions may be skewed because of the restricted sample size. In addition, the format of the study is clinical and anecdotal. Because of the small sample size, and because of the technical difficulties of doing psychotherapy research, the outcomes described here focus on individual case material. Such material cannot furnish "proof" of a clinical or theoretical hypothesis, but can only illustrate and provide examples of clinical observations. It remains for the reader to determine whether such data are consistent with his or her own experience, and are convincing and useful.

Two broad categories of outcome can be described in the psychotherapeutic work with the schizophrenic patients described in this book. The first concerns what I have called the "fundamental practical goal" which consists of helping patients put their thoughts and feelings into words. Verbal psychotherapy of whatever kind cannot occur without such a capacity, and for many schizophrenic patients this function is disturbed at the outset. The traditional techniques of psychotherapy (i.e., clarification, confrontation, and interpretation) cannot function unless the patient is able to communicate a coherent theme to the therapist. If the patient's acting out disrupts the therapeutic setting, or if his use of verbal symbols is disordered, the therapist is not emotionally or cognitively in a position to understand him. Often the therapist must work actively to help create what we take for granted in working with neurotic patients: a setting in which the patient is able to use coherent speech to communicate about his inner states. Accomplishing this task leads to greater conceptualization and socialization of thought, and to the development of insight.

The other outcome one can examine concerns changes in the quality of the patient's object relations, his integration of aggression, his capacity to tolerate affects such as emptiness, despair, envy, loneliness, sadness, and longing for contact. Success in this area involves a working through of schizoid withdrawal. It also involves a reduction of the patient's defensive need to use denial to block out external reality, especially his awareness of the interpersonal aspects of reality and his internal feeling states. Such changes strengthen his ability to appreciate the social criteria of reality (Kernberg, 1975), and thus reality testing in general.

INCREASED CAPACITY TO USE WORDS AND CONCEPTS

As noted in chapter 4, the use of naming and enlargement helped many patients to improve their capacity to put their feelings and thoughts into words. Insofar as these patients had deconceptualized their thinking by means of perceptualization or sensationalization, or had translated concepts into action, rather than ideas or affects, this seemed to lead to at least some reconstitution of conceptual thought.

Some patients recovered concepts and affects which seemed "hidden" in somatic sensations. Mr. DeVito, who had experienced a painful sensation in his throat, was eventually able to connect it with the affect of loneliness. Similarly, he was able to understand that the sensation of having "a hollow in (his) abdomen" was associated with the feeling of emptiness. Later, he was able to elaborate further, describing his inner state as being like "a barren chasm where no human comes in" and like "a deep cave with colorless walls."

At the beginning of psychotherapy, Ms. Weiss literally felt that her mind had calcified. She experienced this as a kind of sensation, and believed that something was wrong with her neurologically (an extensive neurologic workup was negative). Gradually, she was able to connect this sensation with the inner realm of thought and feeling in which she felt emotionally blocked, dead, and empty.

Some patients came to recognize ideas and affect which had been previously perceptualized. As noted earlier, Ms. Bender had experienced Dr. M being intrusive and grating in the form of a visual image of abrasive sandpaper. She was finally able to connect that visual image with her emotional response to him. Ms. Chen was able to link the perception that her therapist was pinching her ear with tweezers with the emotional experience of being controlled. Eventually, this extremely guarded and concrete woman was able to reveal a more vulnerable and emotional side when she described herself as a desolate and fruitless orchard.

Other patients began to understand the link between symptomatic actions which had been substituted for an awareness of their inner states. Before one hospitalization, Mr. Martin had lit a massive fire in his fireplace during the summer because he felt his relatives had given him the "cold shoulder." Eventually, he was able to describe the frigidness of the emotional climate in his family. Ms. Williams had entered the hospital talking gibberish and was later able to acknowledge that this protected her against her feelings of vulnerability and shame. Mr. Tilden was able to recognize that his manner of thinking and speaking in private (rather than publicly shared) phrases served to protect him from rejection and pain. Ms. Williams' propensity for action, especially for getting into fights, gradually diminished as her capacity to identify her inner life developed. This initially impulsive and inarticulate woman was eventually able to say, "I don't feel human when I'm all alone. It's like an immense expanse of nothingness." She added, "Feeling homesick is like a wound, not an actual wound, but a wound in my feelings."

It appears that the reversing of deconceptualization leads to a resocialization of thinking. Thinking emerges from a private conceptional world and once again is connected to the public, shared world of class concepts. The patient can begin to use culturally shared concepts and can more easily link himself to the inner lives of others. For example, Mr. Tindel used a private language in which "couch," "fireplace," "sunny," and "music" meant "soothing." He felt that his ideas wandered around as if they had lost their way and were no longer connected to the outside world. He and his therapist eventually were able to discuss ways in which such private conceptions and "half-thoughts" helped Mr. Tilden to protect himself from the full impact of feelings and from the fear of relating to others.

As mentioned earlier, Ms. Williams also used private thinking and speech to create a protective wall between herself and others. "The statements I make," she said, "are so that people won't know what I'm feeling." Ms. Hunt used rapid speech filled with private connections to avoid contact with others. What in both cases appeared phenomenologically to be profound looseness of association, proved to be at least somewhat remediable. In both cases, the patient learned to use public concepts rather than private images and became far more comprehensible.

Once the patient has access to shared cultural symbols (i.e., class concepts) a "calculus" of conceptual thinking can develop. On the simplest level, one concept can be associatively linked to another. These links are no longer established on the basis of physical or temporal contiguity, or concrete perceptual or sensory similarity which had previously linked more concrete images. Links based on contiguity are the basis of primary process and concrete thinking (Freud, 1900) and what Vygotsky (1934) referred to as thinking in congeries, complexes, or pseudoconcepts. In truly conceptual thinking, links are established on the basis of a similarity in the form of *concepts*, rather than of concrete sensory images. It seems that these kinds of links spontaneously lead to the formation of analogy and metaphor.[1]

In symbolic logic (Langer, 1967), analogy refers to a similarity of *form* between two phenomena. One form may be used to stand for or symbolize another. *Metaphor* is a closely related linguistic structure. Metaphor points to an analogy between two forms from different frames of reference (technically, different "universes of discourse"). When a poet compares his lover's sparkling eyes to twinkling stars, he is equating two similar forms (radiance) from different frames of reference. Metaphor expands our cognitive lexicon by asking us to look beyond conventional

---

[1]One may speak of a primitive and concrete type of analogy, such as the infant's awareness of the similarity between the shape of a crescent moon and a banana This kind of analogy is the basis for primitive unconscious symbols such as phallic symbols. It consists of a recognition of similarity in simple perceptual or sensory experience. In the above discussion, analogy refers to a similarity in the form of culturally shared class concepts. This involves a recognition of similarities between experience distant or "abstract" concepts.

associations and to see new meanings highlighted by new frames of reference (Ricoeur, 1976). The poet realizes, for example, that, like stars, his lover's eyes seem ethereal, magical, and brilliant.

It appears that once abstract class concepts have been generated, the linking of such class concept elements via analogy and metaphor becomes much easier, and, at times, seems to proceed spontaneously.[2] This expands the realm of conceptual, rather than concrete thought.

When Dr. C missed an appointment due to an illness, Ms. Williams, the formerly inarticulate 20-year-old, said, "Well, I felt like you deserted me. Like you deserted the ship." Her metaphor of the ship implied a camaraderie with a crew and a trip with a destination, suggesting the existence of an alliance as well as hopefulness despite her disappointment. In discussing her feeling, she commented: "Missing people is like a wound, not a physical wound, but a mental wound."

Mr. DeVito described his sense of isolation and longing for others. It was, he said, "like being in a glass jar, and being unable to get out." In describing his sense of loss and the feeling that he had no value, he said: "It was as if I dropped a hundred diamonds from a cliff, and watched them vanish into the sea." In portraying his tendency to withdraw into silence during conversations, he said, "Silences are like a dungeon in which I stay cut off from others."

Ms. Williams commented on her missing a friend who was being discharged from the hospital, "I feel like my heart is being ripped out of me." This somatic metaphor seems to border on frank sensationalization of thought. One can easily imagine that such a metaphor might become the basis of a deconceptualized somatic sensation of heart pain. At this point, Ms. Williams was more able to tolerate her affect states, and she was consciously drawing a comparison between heart pain and pain in the sphere of an inner emotional realm. The pain in her emotional universe was no longer sensationalized as sensory pain.[3]

---

[2]Certainly, without the building blocks of concepts, abstract conceptual thought is impossible. There are no concepts to organize or compare, there are no ideas to think "about." Thinking, even if it were potentially possible, would have no elements to act upon. According to Bion (1957), thinking evolves to deal with thoughts.

[3]Certain emotions may actually be associated with certain physiologic states: emotional hurt or lonesomeness with pain in the heart, anxiety with dizziness, rage with a sensation of heat. When thought becomes concrete, the realm of affect collapses and

The metaphors described above represent thinking which has emerged from schizophrenic concreteness. These statements implicitly acknowledge an inner psychic life which can be described by comparing it to analogous physical phenomena. But, the distinction between the psychic and the physical is preserved. Physical reality serves as an analogy to mental and emotional life; it is not an equivalent.

The spontaneous development of insight is closely connected with the development of analogy and metaphor. According to modern symbolic logic (Langer, 1967), insight is considered to be an intuitive capacity to see equivalent forms in different phenomena.[4] In psychology, insight might be described as the capacity to recognize equivalent forms in psychological, emotional, or behavioral life. As with analogy and metaphor, once class concepts are more available, the process of comparing them, contrasting them, and organizing them more readily appears. All the patients discussed in this book spontaneously began to make such cognitive links and to attach meaning to these comparisons.

Ms. Williams talked about missing her friends in the hospital, and how lonely she would feel when she left. She recognized a similar "emotional form" in her past. She said with genuine surprise, "You know, this is why I used crack on the outside. I felt lonely and like I had no one to talk to. Like when my uncle died. I felt terrible. It was awful. We went to the wake." Later, she added, "I think this is why I used crack. I think it was to get away from my feelings." Still later, in discussing a relative who emigrated to Mexico, she said, "I feel really bad. This is what caused me to smoke crack. Feeling like this is how come I used (drugs)."

The evolution of analogy, metaphor, and psychological insight described above seems to reverse the regressive path I have hypothesized from concept to perception and sensation that underlies hallucinations and concrete thinking. Patients who begin by experiencing uncanny perceptions and sensations appear to progress by means of naming and enlargement to the use of class concepts and, finally, analogy and metaphor. It is only at this

---

becomes replaced entirely by the sensations which were previously only physiologic accompaniments.

[4]Recognizing the similarity between a spiral staircase and the structure of DNA is, for example, an insight.

point that insight, as defined above, is possible and this can emerge spontaneously. Concepts, the building blocks of insight, are generated at first by the capacity to name. It is the development of this capacity which is the "fundamental practical goal" of psychotherapy with schizophrenic patients, and which the techniques described in this book most immediately aim to achieve.

INCREASED SELF-REVELATION

Once patients developed a willingness and capacity to put their inner experience into words, certain characteristic themes emerged in their psychotherapies.

Revealing Feelings of Emptiness, Deadness, and Rage

Most of the patients described in this book experienced a painful sense of inner deadness and emptiness. We recall that Mr. DeVito described himself as a barren chasm and Ms. Weiss experienced that her mind had calcified. Ms. Williams reported feeling a "vast, empty void" within her. Ms. Jackson and Ms. Chen suffered from a similar feeling of hollowness. The feeling of emptiness and associated experience of deadness was a very characteristic feature of the inner lives of these patients.

Nancy Morgan was a 25-year-old woman with a history of auditory hallucinations, paranoid ideas, grandiose delusions, and social isolation. There was no prominent history of affective symptoms. She had been preoccupied since her early teens, when she first became ill, with concrete concerns about medication issues; for example, when to take her pills and what dose to take. After about six months of psychotherapy, she was able to put her feelings of despair into words, feelings which she had previously pushed out of her awareness. She wept and said, "Nothing will make any difference. I'll never be like other people. I'll never get married, I'll never have children. I'll never do anything useful. There's nothing inside that anyone would ever want to get to know or love. I'll always be alone."

One of the most difficult aspects of psychotherapy for these patients is the effort to put feelings of despair into words. A great

deal of suffering and hopelessness is connected with the experience of emptiness and deadness. Many of these patients would
much prefer to hallucinate, hold onto delusions, or behave bizarrely than to confront the absence of self-feeling. The focus of
much of the psychotherapy is to help the patient, "Stop, look,
and listen" (Semrad, Menaer, Mann, and Standish, 1952; Semrad,
1966) and turn conscious attention to these feeling states.

Interestingly, there appeared to be a rather strong connection between these experiences and a powerful rage which was
split off and denied. When the psychotherapy was able to help
the patient feel more conscious anger and destructiveness, the
patient often felt more alive, more vigorous, and more real.

For many years, Mr. DeVito had felt isolated, dead, inert,
and formless. He felt little inner vitality, purpose, or initiative.
Gradually, he began to feel more able to express his annoyance
and, finally, rage at his cousin, whom he felt had always been
disrespectful. This culminated in a yelling match at a local bar.
He was also able at this time to get more angry with Dr. B and
expressed the wish to smash Dr. B with his fists. He had a dream
of murdering a man who appeared to be a thinly disguised version
of his therapist. The expression of these feelings was frightening,
but also seemed quite liberating. Mr. DeVito's sense of deadness
began, slowly, to lift. "I feel like I'm having my natural feelings
now. I didn't put the brakes on with my cousin. I feel like I'm a
real person." For the first time, he said, he felt like he had a center
and was not so unclear about what his feelings were. He did not
feel so confused about what to say in social situations.

Ms. Weiss talked about a long-standing feeling of inner lifelessness. Virtually nothing could change it. Therapy sessions were
filled with a sense of torpor, apathy, and nothingness. Dr. E suggested that her inner lifelessness might be a way of shutting herself down so that she could not harm anyone with her rage.
Usually, this interpretation did not produce much change.

Rather suddenly, Ms. Weiss began to talk about violent and
murderous wishes. She wanted to blow up the state capitol and
kill the governor. She felt out of control and was worried that she
might want to hurt Dr. E. During this time, Ms. Weiss seemed
more animated, more activated, and more alive, even though
tense and extremely frightened about her "raving" and being
"on a rampage." As quickly as they had come, her fantasies of

murder and violence vanished. Once again, she returned to her customary torpor. It seemed to her therapist that she had disarmed herself by dismantling her executive apparatus. In such a state she could neither blow up buildings, nor harm anyone. Unlike neurotic patients who might do and undo certain actions linked to aggression, Ms. Weiss's defensive behavior appeared to take place on a more rudimentary level of the executive ego. In effect, the entire ego apparatus was put out of action. Ms. Weiss hinted at such a mechanism when she said at one point, "My mind doesn't work well enough for me to get mad." In a similar vein, Mr. Tilden commented, "There are pressures in my mind that block me from thinking."

Revealing the Sense of a Damaged or Destroyed Self

Most of the patients described in this book experienced either an extremely fragile or a nonexistent sense of self. The more patients became able to report their inner states, the more they reported a disturbance in their sense of self. Mr. DeVito complained bitterly of an "absence of self" and felt that he had nothing to say in conversations because there was no center to his personality. Ms. Chen often felt "fractured" and that her body was vulnerable to manipulation and attack. Mr. Tilden also felt "splintered" by interactions with others, and felt extremely vulnerable to a painful sense of intrusion and control.

Frequently, patients reported that they needed to maintain a secret and protected place where the "self" could exist safe from criticism, intrusion, coercion, or attack. Mr. Tilden said that he sometimes felt like "a turtle" who "hid under his shell" from people who could "splinter" him. Ms. Chen spoke of a "personal space" which people would intrude upon at the risk of her explosive anger. These reports are reminiscent of Winnicott's formulation (1960a) concerning the defensive function of a false self that protects the true self which has been secreted away.

Mr. DeVito discussed his fragmentary sense of personal identity and said that perhaps he avoided a more definite knowledge of his feelings and thus a more definite identity in order to escape retaliation for his destructiveness. Mr. Tilden revealed that he was afraid to assume a more certain identity because he felt it would be too confining. He said, "I can't decide what job to take. If I picked one, and didn't pick another, I would feel like I was being drowned or smothered. It would be like being locked in a closet." Searles (1979) reported something similar in the schizophrenic patients he worked with. He believed that some of his patients were afraid to consolidate their sense of identity for fear that they would be confined or suffocated by the limits of any self-definition they might adopt.

Some patients feel that psychotherapy entices them to "come out" of a fantasy or dream world and prods them to enter the harsher, colder "real" world. This can feel enormously unsafe and threatening. Patients may feel discouraged, painfully lonely, and bewildered by all the demands of everyday life. They may feel sapped of all their energy, as if unplugged from a source of security and animation in the world of fantasy. Mr. Tilden "came out of (his) cocoon" only to feel a debilitating lassitude. He said, "No one cares, no one calls. There was nothing for me in my cocoon, and there is nothing for me out here." He went on, "Being optimistic in my fantasy cocoon was easy. Being optimistic in the real world is not."

Mr. DeVito expressed similar feelings about going out into the world. He had several dreams that linked living apart from his relatives with the possibility of sexual relations with women, and exciting adventures. Nevertheless, each time he tried to live separately, his sense of loneliness in a world utterly indifferent to his presence felt intolerable. In order to escape these painful feelings, he spent much of the day sleeping.

DECREASED DENIAL

As noted in chapter 1, many writers believe that the denial of external reality is a building block of psychotic structure. Denial of external perceptions, of social conventions about what is real, and of inner affective states, plays a large role in psychotic functioning. In the realm of the internal world, denial wards off excruciating affects such as emptiness, deadness, a sense of being inhuman and monstrous, and loss. In the realm of the external world, denial wards off perceptions and impressions, which are linked to meanings that can generate intolerable emotions.

Perhaps with the exception of paranoid reactions, denial is the psychological phenomenon most resistant to change in psychotherapy. It leads to a massive and far-reaching change in the balance of mental forces. When external reality and internal affect can be escaped, all kinds of psychotic anxiety-reducing psychological adaptations become possible.

The techniques described in this book seem to have helped at least some of the patients to reduce their use of denial. Some examples of greater recognition and sharing of painful feelings have already been given. I will describe another.

Mr. Tilden had not worked in months. He spent a lot of time thinking about his future and what kind of career he wanted. He wondered if he should become a musician. Similarly, he wondered if he should become an actor. He put great stock in these possibilities, despite having no experience or training in either. These options seem disconnected from any material evidence of talent or commitment. At the same time, the patient angrily rejected jobs which he considered beneath him. It is characteristic of some schizophrenic patients that they reject undemanding work, which they consider too simple and demeaning, but tenaciously hold onto plans for careers requiring talents and abilities, which there is little evidence that they have.

Mr. Douglas, a 25-year-old schizophrenic man who had completed two years of college, but who had not been able to keep a job, said maybe he would pursue a career as a sports broadcaster. Maybe he would take classes in the spring. He asked if he should pursue a career in radio announcing. After some discussion, his therapist said, "I don't quite understand why you would plan a career as a sportscaster, when you have not done any work in radio. You have not taken any classes, and have not had an apprenticeship." The patient became furious. The therapist only wanted to crush his dreams and make him feel worthless. After more discussion of feelings of embarrassment, hurt, and sadness, the patient was able to acknowledge how painful it was to feel he was less skilled and talented than others, and that while he might have talent as an announcer, nothing he had done so far would justify choosing broadcasting as a career.

In work with psychotic patients, one sometimes comes to a point where it seems that a crossroads is reached. Split-off delusional beliefs collide with a more and more competent and adaptive ego. Such a moment can have a curious, topsy-turvy quality where the figure and ground of psychosis and health wrestle for supremacy. The psychotherapy of Mr. DeVito provides an example. He had been hospitalized twice in quick succession. It was not exactly clear what had precipitated these hospitalizations. One factor seemed to be the patient's paranoid fears of returning, after his first hospital stay, to the neighborhood where he lived. Another appeared to be his recent attempt to live in an apartment apart from his aunt that had left him feeling lonely and shaky.

For some time Dr. B, his therapist, had emphasized how important it was for the patient to be able to function at work. This had a certain sense to it in that when he wasn't working, Mr. DeVito became more and more withdrawn. At such times he stopped functioning as an adult, and became a kind of "lump." Self-esteem based on his real world achievements, of which there were several, seemed to fade into oblivion, and could not help support his efforts to assert himself and succeed. Work had always seemed to be an island of healthy adaptation which anchored him in the real rather than the regressive world.

In any case, despite Dr. B's encouragement to return to his bank job (which the patient had worked at with success for five years), he decompensated repeatedly. He became paranoid and delusional and was holed up in his room. The patient insisted during these episodes that he was not crazy and that he was simply "taking a rest." On another occasion he took a ferry to an island off the Oregon coast where he barely survived—he was discovered and rescued by a park ranger. He insisted that this had nothing to do with being ill, but was, instead, a "voyage of self-discovery." He said, "I don't want anyone calling me sick. I am not sick. There is no way I'm sick."

After his second hospitalization, the patient raised the issue of insurance coverage with Dr. B. He asked Dr. B to talk with the medical benefits officer at his bank so that he could be reimbursed for his hospital stay. Dr. B pointed out the contradiction in what the patient was doing. On the one hand, he insisted that his locking himself in his room and his trip to the Oregon island were not a result of illness and insisted that he was not sick. On the other he wanted medical experts (including Dr. B) to certify that he was entitled to benefits because of illness. The patient gave an unguarded laugh and said, "I'm in a tough spot, I guess. I really got myself in a jam. I need the money. I'll have to think this one over." Over time, the patient began to think more seriously about his "illness." To acknowledge his illness for him was to acknowledge that he was "crazy." When he was finally able to consider this possibility seriously, he wept inconsolably.

THE DEEPENING OF OBJECT RELATIONS

Many of the patients who participated in psychotherapy for an extended period of time became more able to become involved in other human relationships. They were more able to seek contact, to ask for help, to acknowledge the importance of others, to tolerate delay and frustration, to risk and to reveal themselves to others. By and large, they were better able to avoid the temptation to break off relationships when loss and pain felt overwhelming.

Ms. Williams had worked with Dr. C for many months in the hospital. When Dr. C told her that she would be leaving, she responded by avoiding several meetings. Finally, she came and talked. Despite her sense of betrayal, pain, and anger, she was committed enough to her relationship with Dr. C to tell her how she had hurt the patient. She said, "I feel like you are walking out on me. Like everyone does." Later on she exclaimed, "To hell with you. I wish you were a can I could crush." A short time later, the patient told Dr. C, "When you go (from the unit), I'll feel alone and sad. They'll want to give me a new therapist. But it won't be the same. I don't want someone different. I just want to work with you."

What was impressive was that for most of her life, Ms. Williams had translated painful affect almost immediately into action. She had distracted herself with cocaine and affected the pose of a devil-may-care gang member. During the later stages of her hospital treatment, she was able to tolerate sadness and loss, and to put those affects into words. Moreover, she was able to acknowledge that Dr. C was someone important to her, who could not be summarily replaced. All this was accompanied by great inner pain.

Mr. Tilden often appeared to pursue his own thoughts. He got caught up in elaborate fantasies and disconnected ruminating. He expressed great scorn for his therapist, Dr. T. When Dr. T asked about this, he became enraged. He insisted on changing the subject. Nevertheless, Dr. T persisted, and Mr. Tilden experienced her as attacking and controlling, in an effort to destroy him. He felt accused of being a sinister person. Finally he wept, and said that it was true, he did have a destructive side. He also acknowledged that he needed the therapist to support him and help calm him, and that to admit this made him feel frightened, vulnerable, and exposed.

Mr. Tilden was able to tolerate frustration, suspiciousness, fear of attack, and pain well enough to refrain from discarding his therapist as an enemy. He was able to acknowledge unpleasant feelings, and to maintain an image of Dr. T as someone who was at least somewhat valuable. Mr. Tilden's temptation to dismiss Dr. T in a paranoid rage was great.

Along with an increase in these patients' capacities to establish a relationship with the therapist, were improved interpersonal functioning in their lives outside therapy. Mr. Tilden developed a number of friendships which actually helped him feel less isolated and alone for the first time in his life. Also for the first time, he began to have some sexual contact with women. After years of difficulty concentrating and functioning at work, he was able to perform well at a job, which required considerable interpersonal skills, over a period of several years.

Ms. Chen, who had been a virtual isolate since childhood, was able to develop a romantic relationship with a man which lasted almost a year. While this relationship stirred up intense emotions which ultimately led to its breakup, still Ms. Chen's willingness and ability to remain connected this durably was a genuine step forward. Ms. Chen, who felt that the preservation of her "personal space" was a matter of survival, had been able to spend long weekends with her boyfriend during their relationship. Before the end of therapy, the patient had weathered several rifts and reconciliations with her boyfriend and gained real experience in being intimate.

Ms. Williams became aware of a need for other people which seemed not to have existed before. When she first began psychotherapy, Ms. Williams was physically intimidating and bizarre. She had little contact with her own emotional life, and was not aware of the impact of her actions on others. Her peers on the unit kept their distance. When her psychotherapy ended, she was able to feel sadness, loneliness, and affection in much greater depth.

Moreover, her fellow patients sought her out to include her in their lives. This meant a great deal to a woman who had felt herself to be a kind of excommunicated monster.

Mr. DeVito had lived with his aunt and uncle for a year, and had not had a relationship with a woman since college. Over the course of his psychotherapy, he was able to maintain several friendships with his male friends, and establish significant relationships with several woman. He dated one woman for several years who ultimately wanted to marry him. The relationship broke up, perhaps because the patient was frightened of this degree of intimacy. Still, Mr. DeVito had allowed himself to make a powerful bond with someone outside his family for the first time in almost fifteen years. Despite the breakup of this romance, Mr. DeVito did not retreat to his former isolation, but after a time, was willing to try relationships with other women.

References

American Psychiatric Association (1980), *Diagnostic and Statistical Manual of Mental Disorders*, 3rd ed. (DSM-III). Washington, DC: American Psychiatric Press.

———— (1987), *Diagnostic and Statistical Manual of Mental Disorders*, 3rd ed. rev. (DSM-III-R). Washington, DC: American Psychiatric Press.

Andreason, N. (1985), Positive vs. negative schizophrenia: A critical re-evaluation. *Schizophr. Bull.*, 11:380–389.

Angyl, A. (1944), Disturbances of thinking in schizophrenia. In: *Language and Thought in Schizophrenia*, ed. J. Kasanin. New York: W. W. Norton, pp. 115–123.

Arieti, S. (1974), *The Interpretation of Schizophrenia*. New York: Basic Books.

Arlow, J. (1980), The genesis of interpretation. In: *Psychoanalytic Explorations of Technique: Discourse on the Theory of Therapy*, ed. H. Blum. New York: International Universities Press, pp. 193–206.

———— Brenner, C. (1964), The psychopathology of the psychoses. In: *Psychoanalytic Concepts and the Structural Theory*. New York: International Universities Press, pp. 144–178.

———— ———— (1969), The psychopathology of the psychoses: A proposed revision. *Internat. J. Psycho-Anal.*, 50:5–14.

Auchincloss, E., & Weiss, R. (1992), Paranoid character and the intolerance of indifference. *J. Amer. Psychoanal. Assn.*, 40:1013–1037.

Bak, R. (1954), The schizophrenic defense against aggression. *Internat. J. Psycho-Anal.*, 35:129–134.

Balint, M. (1959), Regression in the analytic situation. In: *Thrills and Regression*. New York: International Universities Press.

Bartlett, J., Ed. (1980), *Familiar Quotations. A Collection of Passages, Phrases, and Proverbs Traced to Their Sources in Ancient and Modern Literature*, 15th ed. ed E.M. Beck. Boston: Little Brown and Company.

Baxter, L. Jr., Schwartz, J., Berman, K., Szuba, M., Guze, B., Mazziota, J., Alazraki, A., Selin, C., Ferng, H., Munford, P., & Phelps, M. (1992), Caudate glucose metabolic rate changes with both drug and behavior therapy for obsessive compulsive disorder. *Arch. Gen. Psychiatry*, 49:681–689.

Bellack, A., Mueser, K., Morrison, R., Tierney, A., & Podell, K. (1990), Remediation of cognitive deficits in schizophrenia. *Amer. J. Psychiatry*, 147:1650–1655.

Benedek, T. (1959), Parenthood as a developmental phase: A contribution to libido theory. *J. Amer. Psychoanal. Assn.*, 7:389–417.

Beres, D., & Arlow, J. (1974), Fantasy and identification in empathy. *Psychoanal. Quart.*, 43:26–50.

Bergman, A. (1982), Considerations about development of the girl during the separation individuation process. In: *Early Female Development*, ed. D. Mendell. New York: Spectrum Publications, pp. 61–80.

Bion, W. R. (1956), Development of schizophrenic thought. In: *Second Thoughts: Selected Papers on Psychoanalysis*. New York: Basic Books, 1967, pp. 36–42.

――― (1957), Differentiation of the psychotic from the non-psychotic personalities. In: *Second Thoughts: Selected Papers on Psychoanalysis*. New York: Basic Books, 1967, pp. 43–64.

――― (1959), Attacks on linking. *Internat. J. Psycho-Anal.*, 40:93–109.

Bleuler, E. (1911), *Dementia Praecox or the Group of Schizophrenias*, tr. J. Ziakin. New York: International Universities Press, 1960.

Boyer, L. B., & Giovachini, P. (1967), *Psychoanalytic Treatment of Characterological and Schizophrenic Disorders*. New York: Science House.

――― ――― (1980), *Psychoanalytic Treatment of Schizophrenic, Borderline and Characterological Disorders*, 2nd ed. New York: Jason Aronson.

Brenner, C. (1980), Working alliance, therapeutic alliance and transference. In: *Psychoanalytic Explorations of Technique: Discourse on the Theory of Therapy*, ed. H. Blum. New York: International Universities Press.

Breuer, J., & Freud, S. (1895), Studies on Hysteria. *Standard Edition*, 2. London: Hogarth Press, 1955.

Burnham, D. L. (1955), Some problems in communication with schizophrenic patients. *J. Amer. Psychoanal. Assn.*, 3:67–81.

Bychowski, G. (1957), From latent to manifest schizophrenia. *Congress Report, 2nd International Congress for Psychiatry* (Zurich), 3:128–134.

Carpenter, W. T. (1984), Perspectives on the psychotherapy of schizophrenia project. *Schizophr. Bull.*, 10:599–603.

――― Strauss, J. S., & Bartko, J. J. (1973), Flexible system for the diagnosis of schizophrenia: Report from the WHO international pilot study of schizophrenia. *Science*, 182:1275–1278.

Clark, L. P. (1933), Treatment of narcissistic neuroses and psychoses. *Psychoanal. Quart.*, 20:304–326.

Clifft, M. (1986), Writing about psychiatric patients, guidelines for disguising case material. *Bull. Menninger Clinic*, 50:511–524.

Davis, M., & Fernald, R. (1990), Social control of neuronal soma size. *J. Neurol.*, 21:1180–1188.

Eissler, K. (1953a), The effects of structure of the ego on psychoanalytic technique. *J. Amer. Psychoanal. Assn.*, 1:104–143.

——— (1953b), Notes upon the emotionality of a schizophrenic patient and its relation to problems of technique. *The Psychoanalytic Study of the Child*, 8:199–251. New York: International Universities Press.

——— (1954), Notes upon defects of ego structure in schizophrenia. *Internat. J. Psycho-Anal.*, 35:141–146.

Fairbairn, W. R. D. (1941), A revised psychology of the psychoses and psychoneuroses. *Internat. J. Psycho-Anal.*, 22:250–279.

——— (1944), Endopsychic structure considered in terms of object relationships. *Internat. J. Psycho-Anal.*, 25:70–93.

Farah, M. (1988), Is visual imagery really visual? Overlooked evidence from neuropsychology. *Psychol. Rev.*, 95:307–317.

——— (1989), The neural basis of mental imagery. *Trends Neurosci.*, 12:395–399.

Federn, P. (1934), The analysis of psychotics. *Internat. J. Psycho-Anal.*, 15:209–214.

——— (1943a), Psychoanalysis of the psychoses. I. Errors and how to avoid them. *Psychiatric Quart.*, 17:3–19.

——— (1943b), Psychoanalysis of the psychoses. II. Transference. *Psychiatric Quart.*, 17:240–257.

——— (1943c), Psychoanalysis of the psychoses. III. The psychoanalytic process. *Psychiatric Quart.*, 17:470–487.

——— (1952), *Ego Psychology and the Psychoses*, ed. E. Weiss. New York: Basic Books.

Feighner, J. P., Robins, E., Guze, S. B., Woodruff, R., Winokur, G., & Munoz, R. (1972), Diagnostic criteria for use in psychiatric research. *Arch. Gen. Psychiatry*, 26:57–63.

Fenichel, O. (1945), *The Psychoanalytic Theory of the Neuroses*. New York: W. W. Norton.

Fernald, R. (1993), Cichlids in love. *The Sciences, Essays and Comment*, July, Aug.: 27–31, ed. Peter Brown. New York: New York Academy of Sciences.

Frank, A., & Gunderson, J. (1990), The role of the therapeutic alliance in the treatment of schizophrenia: Relationship of course and outcome. *Arch. Gen. Psychiatry*, 47:228–236.

Freud, A. (1962), The theory of the parent–infant relationship, contribution to the discussion. In: *The Writings*, Vol. 5. New York: International Universities Press, 1969.

Freud, S. (1900), The Interpretation of Dreams. *Standard Edition*, 4 & 5. London: Hogarth Press, 1953.

——— (1905), Fragment of an analysis of a case of hysteria. *Standard Edition*, 7:3–122. London: Hogarth Press, 1953.

————— (1911), Psychoanalytic notes on an autobiographical account of a case of paranoia (dementia paranoides). *Standard Edition,* 12:3–79. London: Hogarth Press, 1958.

————— (1912), Recommendations to physicians practicing psycho-analysis. *Standard Edition,* 12:109–120. London: Hogarth Press, 1958.

————— (1914), On narcissism: An introduction. *Standard Edition,* 14:69–102. London: Hogarth Press, 1957.

————— (1915), The unconscious. *Standard Edition,* 14:161–204. London: Hogarth Press, 1957.

————— (1916–1917), Introductory Lectures on Psychoanalysis. *Standard Edition,* 16. London: Hogarth Press, 1963.

————— (1921), Group psychology and the analysis of the ego. *Standard Edition,* 18:67–143. London: Hogarth Press, 1955.

————— (1923), The ego and the id. *Standard Edition,* 19:3–59. London: Hogarth Press, 1961.

————— (1924a), Neurosis and psychosis. *Standard Edition,* 19:149–153. London: Hogarth Press, 1961.

————— (1924b), The loss of reality in neurosis and psychosis. *Standard Edition,* 19:183–187. London: Hogarth Press, 1961.

————— (1925), Negation. *Standard Edition,* 19:235–239. London: Hogarth Press, 1961.

————— (1927), Fetishism. *Standard Edition,* 21:152–157. London: Hogarth Press, 1961.

————— (1930), Civilization and its discontents. *Standard Edition,* 21:59–145. London: Hogarth Press, 1961.

————— (1937), Analysis terminable and interminable. *Standard Edition,* 23:216–253. London: Hogarth Press, 1964.

————— (1940), An outline of psychoanalysis. *Standard Edition,* 23:144–207. London: Hogarth Press, 1964.

Fromm-Reichmann, F. (1959), *Psychoanalysis and Psychotherapy: Selected Papers.* Chicago: University of Chicago Press.

Frosch, J. (1964), The psychotic character: Clinical psychiatric consideration. *Psychiatric Quart.,* 38:81–96.

Glass, L., Katz, H., Schnitzer, R., Knapp, P., Frank, A., & Gunderson, J. (1989), Psychotherapy of schizophrenia: An empirical investigation of the relationship of process to outcome. *Amer. J. Psychiatry,* 146:603–608.

Glover, E. (1955), *The Technique of Psychoanalysis.* New York: International Universities Press.

Goldstein, K. (1944), Methodological approach to the study of schizophrenic thought disorder. In: *Language, Thought and Schizophrenia,* ed. J. Kasanin. New York: W. W. Norton, pp. 17–39.

Greenacre, P. (1958), Early psychic determinates of a sense of identity. *J. Amer. Psychoanal. Assn.,* 6:612–627.

Greenson, R. (1967), *The Technique and Practice of Psychoanalysis: Volume 1.* New York: International Universities Press.

———— (1968), Disidentifying from mother. *Internat. J. Psycho-Anal.,* 49:370–374.

Gunderson, J., Frank, A., Katz, H., Vanicellia, M., Frosch, J., & Knapp, P. (1984), Effects of psychotherapy in schizophrenia: II, Comparative outcome of two forms of treatment. *Schizophr. Bull.,* 10:564–598.

Harding, C., Brooks, G., Ashikaja, T., Strauss, J., & Breier, A. (1987a), The Vermont longitudinal study of persons with severe mental illness, I: Methodology, study sample and overall status 32 years later. *Amer. J. Psychiatry,* 144:718–726.

———— ———— ———— ———— ———— (1987b), The Vermont longitudinal study of persons with severe mental illness, II: Long term outcome of subjects who retrospectively met DSM-III criteria for schizophrenia. *Amer. J. Psychiatry,* 144:727–735.

Hartmann, H. (1949), Notes on the theory of aggression. *The Psychoanalytic Study of the Child,* 3/4:9–36. New York: International Universities Press.

———— (1953), Contributing to the metapsychology of schizophrenia. In: *Essays on Ego Psychology: Selected Problems in Psychoanalytic Theory.* New York: International Universities Press, 1964, pp. 182–206.

Hawk, A., Carpenter, W., & Strauss, J. (1975), Diagnostic criteria and five year outcome in schizophrenia: A report from the international pilot study of schizophrenia. *Arch. Gen. Psychiatry,* 32:343–347.

Heimann, P. (1950), On countertransference. *Internat. J. Psycho-Anal.,* 31:81–84.

Hirsch, S., & Hollender, M. (1969), Hysterical psychosis: Classification of the concept. *Amer. J. Psychiatry,* 125:909–915.

Hoffer, E. (1950), Reconsideration of Freud's concept of "primary narcissism." Typescript.

Hollender, M., & Hirsch, S. (1964), Hysterical psychosis. *Amer. J. Psychiatry,* 120:1066–1074.

Jacobson, E. (1954), Contributions to the metapsychology of psychotic identifications. *J. Amer. Psychoanal. Assn.,* 2:239–262.

———— (1957), Denial and repression. *J. Amer. Psychoanal. Assn.,* 5:61–92.

———— (1964), *The Self and the Object World.* New York: International Universities Press.

———— (1967), *Psychotic Conflict and Reality.* New York: International Universities Press.

Jensen, T., Bnefke, I., Hyldebrandt, N., Pedersen, H., Petersen, H., & Weile, B. (1982), Cerebral atrophy in young torture victims. *N. Eng. J. Med.,* 307:1341.

Kafka, F. (1925), *The Trial.* New York: Schocken Books, 1935.

Kasanin, J. (1944), The disturbance of conceptual thinking in schizo-phrenia. In: *Language and Thought in Schizophrenia,* ed. J. Kasanin. New York: W. W. Norton, pp. 41–49.

Katan, M. (1954), The importance of the nonpsychotic part of the per-sonality in schizophrenia. *Internat. J. Psycho-Anal.,* 34:119–128.

Kernberg, O. (1970), A psychoanalytic classification of character pathol-ogy. *J. Amer. Psychoanal. Assn.,* 18:800–823.

—— (1975), *Borderline Conditions and Pathological Narcissism.* New York: Jason Aronson.

—— (1984), *Severe Personality Disorders.* New Haven, CT: Yale Univer-sity Press.

—— Selzer, M., Koenigsberg, H., Carr, A., & Appelbaum, A. (1989), *Psychodynamic Psychotherapy of Borderline Patients.* New York: Basic Books.

Klein, M. (1923), Early analysis. In: *Love, Guilt and Reparation and Other Works, 1921–1945.* New York: Dell, 1977, pp. 85–86.

—— (1930), The importance of symbol formation in the develop-ment of the ego. In: *Love, Guilt and Reparation and Other Works, 1921–1945.* New York: Dell, 1977, pp. 219–232.

—— (1935), A contribution to the psychogenesis of manic-depressive states. In: *Love, Guilt and Reparation and Other Works, 1921–1945.* New York: Dell, 1977, pp. 262–289.

—— (1946), Notes on some schizoid mechanisms. In: *Envy and Grati-tude and Other Works.* New York: Dell, 1977, pp. 1–24.

—— (1957), Envy and gratitude. In: *Envy and Gratitude and Other Works.* New York: Dell, 1977, pp. 177–235.

Kohut, H. (1971), *The Analysis of the Self.* New York: International Univer-sities Press.

Kosslyn, S. (1988), Aspects of a cognitive neuroscience of mental imag-ery. *Science,* 240:1621–1626.

—— Alpert, N., Thompson, W., Maljkovic, V., Weise, S., Chabris, C., Hamilton, S., Rauch, S., & Buonanno, F. (1993), Visual mental imagery activates topographically organized visual cortex: PET in-vestigations. *J. Cognit. Neurosci.,* 5:263–287.

Kraepelin, E. (1902), Dementia praecox. In: *Clinical Psychiatry: A Textbook for Students and Physicians,* 6th ed., tr. A. Diefendorf. New York: Macmillan, 1907.

Kulish, N. (1985), Projective identification: A concept overburdened. *Internat. J. Psychoanal. Psychother.,* 11:79–104.

Lampl-de Groot, J. (1962), Ego ideal and super ego. *The Psychoanalytic Study of the Child,* 17:94–106. New York: International Universities Press.

Langer, S. (1967), *An Introduction to Symbolic Logic.* New York: Dover.

Levy, S., & Ninan, P., Eds. (1990), *The Treatment of Acute Psychotic Episodes.* Washington, DC: American Psychiatric Press.

Liberman, R. P., Lillie, F., Falloon, I. R. H., Harpin, R. E., Hutchinson, W., & Stoute, B. (1984), Social skills training with relapsing schizophrenics: An experimental analysis. *Behav. Modif.*, 8:155–179.

———— Massel, H., Most, M., & Wong, S. (1985), Social skills training for chronic mental patients. *Hosp. Comm. Psychiatry*, 36:396–403.

———— Mueser, K., & Wallace, C. (1986), Social skills training for schizophrenia: Individuals at risk for relapse. *Amer. J. Psychiatry*, 143:523–526.

Little, M. (1951), Countertransference and the patient's response to it. *Internat. J. Psycho-Anal.*, 32:32–40.

———— (1957), "R"-the analyst's total response to his patient's needs. *Internat. J. Psycho-Anal.*, 38:240–254.

———— (1958), On delusional transference (transference psychosis). *Internat. J. Psycho-Anal.*, 39:134–138.

Loewald, H. (1980), *Ego and Reality: Papers on Psychoanalysis.* New Haven, CT: Yale University Press.

Lotterman, A. (1987), Psychoanalytic psychotherapy with a hospitalized schizophrenic. In: *Contemporary Psychotherapies*, 2nd ed., ed. G. Belkin. Monterey, CA: Brooks/Cole.

———— (1990), Emotional induction: Communication via the countertransference. *J. Amer. Acad. Psychoanal.*, 18:587–612.

Mahler, M. (1958), Autism and symbiosis. *Internat. J. Psycho-Anal.*, 39:77–83.

———— (1963), Thoughts about development and individuation. *The Psychoanalytic Study of the Child*, 18:307–324. New York: International Universities Press.

———— (1968), *On Human Symbiosis and the Vicissitudes of Individuation.* New York: International Universities Press.

McGuire, P. K., Shah, G. M., & Murray, R. M. (1993), Increased blood flow in Broca's area during auditory hallucinations in schizophrenia. *The Lancet*, 342:703–706.

Morrison, R., & Bellack, A. (1984), Social skills training. In: *Schizophrenia: Treatment Management and Rehabilitation*, ed. A. Bellack. Orlando, FL: Grune & Stratton.

Munich, R. L. (1987), Conceptual trends and issues in the psychotherapy of schizophrenia. *Amer. J. Psychother.*, 41:23–37.

Neziroglu, F., Steele, J., Yaryura-Tobias, J., Hitri, A., & Diamond, B. (1990), Effect of behavior therapy on serotonin level in obsessive-compulsive disorder. In: *Psychiatry: A World Perspective*, Vol. 3, ed. C. N. Stefanis, A. D. Rabavillas, & C. R. Soldatos. New York: Elsevier Science Publishers, B.V. (Biomedical Division), pp. 707–710.

Ninan, P. (1990), Diagnostic issues. In: *Schizophrenia: Treatment of Acute Psychotic Episodes*, ed. S. Levy & P. Ninan. Washington, DC: American Psychiatric Press.

Nunberg, H. (1931), The synthetic function of the ego. *Internat. J. Psycho-Anal.*, 12:123–140.

Ogden, T. (1979), On projective identification. *Internat. J. Psycho-Anal.*, 60:357–373.

—— (1982), *Projective Identification and Psychotherapeutic Technique*. New York: Jason Aronson.

Olinick, S. (1954), Some considerations on the use of questioning as a psychoanalytic technique. *J. Amer. Psychoanal. Assn.*, 2:57–66.

Orwell, G. (1949), *Nineteen Eighty-Four*. New York: Harcourt, Brace, Jovanovich.

Person, E., & Ovesey, L. (1978), Transvestism: New perspectives. *J. Amer. Acad. Psychoanal.*, 6:301–323.

Piaget, J., & Inhelder, B. (1969), *The Psychology of the Child*. New York: Basic Books.

Racker, H. (1968), *Transference and Countertransference*. New York: International Universities Press.

Reich, A. (1954), Early identification as archaic elements in the superego. *J. Amer. Psychoanal. Assn.*, 2:218–238.

Reich, W. (1945), *Character Analysis: Principles and Technique for Psychoanalysts in Practice and Training*. New York: Orgone Institute Press.

Ricoeur, P. (1976), *Interpretation Theory: Discourse and the Surplus of Meaning*. Fort Worth, TX: Texas Christian University Press.

Rosen, J. (1953), *Direct Analysis*. New York: Grune & Stratton.

Rosenfeld, H. (1952), Notes on the psychoanalysis of the superego conflict of an acute schizophrenic patient. *Internat. J. Psycho-Anal.*, 33:111–131.

—— (1954), Considerations regarding the psychoanalytic approach to acute and chronic schizophrenia. *Internat. J. Psycho-Anal.*, 34:135–140.

—— (1965), *Psychotic States: A Psychoanalytic Approach*. New York: International Universities Press.

—— (1969), On the treatment of psychotic states by psychoanalysis: An historical approach. *Internat. J. Psycho-Anal.*, 50:615–631.

—— (1987), *Impasse and Interpretation: Therapeutic and Anti-Therapeutic Factors in the Psychoanalytic Treatment of Psychotic, Borderline and Neurotic Patients*. New York: Tavistock.

Sarti, P., & Cournos, F. (1990), Medication and psychotherapy in the treatment of chronic schizophrenia. *Psychiatric Clin. N.A.*, 13:215–228.

Schafer, R. (1968), *Aspects of Internalization*. New York: International Universities Press.

Schneider, K. (1959), *Clinical Psychopathology*. tr. M. Hamilton. New York: Grune & Stratton.

Searles, H. (1962), The differentiation between concrete and metaphorical thinking in the recovering schizophrenic patient. *J. Amer. Psychoanal. Assn.*, 10:22–49.

——— (1963), Transference psychosis in the psychotherapy of schizophrenia. *Internat. J. Psycho-Anal.*, 44:249–281.

——— (1965), *Collected Papers on Schizophrenia and Related Subjects*. New York: International Universities Press.

——— (1971), Pathological symbiosis and autism. In: *In The Name of Life—Essays in Honor of Eric Fromm*, ed. B. Landis & E. Tauber. New York: Holt, Rinehart & Winston, pp. 69–83.

——— (1972), The function of the patient's realistic perception of the analyst in delusional transference. *Brit. J. Med. Psychol.*, 45:1–18.

——— (1979), *Countertransference and Related Subjects*. New York: International Universities Press.

Segal, H. (1950), Some aspects of the analysis of schizophrenia. *Internat. J. Psycho-Anal.*, 31:268–278.

——— (1964), *Introduction to the Work of Melanie Klein*. New York: Basic Books, 1973.

Semrad, E. (1966), Long term therapy of schizophrenia: Formulation of the clinical approach. In: *Psychoneuroses and Schizophrenia*, ed. G. Usdin. Philadelphia: J. B. Lippincott, pp. 155–173.

——— Menaer, D., Mann, J., & Standish, C. (1952), A study of the doctor–patient relationship in psychotherapy of psychotic patients. *Psychiatry*, 15:377–385.

Shakespeare, W. (c. 1599), *Hamlet*, ed. H Jenkins. New York: Routledge, 1982.

Siomopoulas, V. (1971), Hysterical psychosis: Psychopathological aspects. *Brit. J. Med. Psychol.*, 44:95–100.

Spiegel, D., & Frank, R. (1979), Hysterical psychosis and hypnotizability. *Amer. J. Psychiatry*, 136:777–781.

Spitz, R. (1965), *The First Year of Life: A Psychoanalytic Study of Normal and Deviant Development of Object Relations*. New York: International Universities Press.

Spotnitz, J. (1969), *Modern Psychoanalysis of the Schizophrenic Patient: Theory of the Technique*. New York: Grune & Stratton.

Stanton, A., Gunderson, J., Knapp, P., Frank, A., Vanicellia, M., Schnitzer, R., & Rosenthal, R. (1984), Effects of psychotherapy in schizophrenia: I. Design and implementation of a controlled study. *Schizophr. Bull.*, 10:520–563.

Sterba, R. (1934), The fate of the ego in analytic therapy. *Internat. J. Psycho-Anal.*, 15:117–126.

Stern, D. (1985), *The Interpersonal World of the Infant: A View from Psychoanalysis and Developmental Psychology*. New York: Basic Books.

Stoller, R. (1974), Symbiosis anxiety and the development of masculinity. *Arch. Gen. Psychiatry*, 30:164–172.

Sullivan, H. S. (1940), *Conceptions of Modern Psychiatry*. New York: W. W. Norton.

——— (1953), *The Interpersonal Theory of Psychiatry*. New York: W. W. Norton.

——— (1962), *Schizophrenia as a Human Process*. New York: W. W. Norton.

——— (1964), *The Fusion of Psychiatry and Social Science*. New York: W. W. Norton.

Vaillant, G. (1975), Ten to fifteen year follow-up of remitting schizophrenics. Paper presented at the 128th annual meeting of the American Psychiatric Association, Anaheim, CA, May 5–9.

Vygotsky, L. (1934), *Thought and Language*. Cambridge, MA: MIT Press, 1986.

Waddington, J. C. (1993), Sight and insight: "Visualization" of auditory hallucinations in schizophrenia? *The Lancet*, 342:692–693.

Walder, R. (1925), The psychoses: Their mechanisms and accessibility to influence. *Internat. J. Psycho-Anal.*, 6:259–281.

Weissman, A. (1958), Reality sense and reality testing. *Behav. Sci.*, 3:228–261.

Will, O. (1975), Schizophrenia V: Psychological treatment. In: *The Comprehensive Textbook of Psychiatry*, ed. A. Freedman, H. Kaplan, & B. Sadock. Baltimore: Williams & Wilkins.

Winnicott, D. W. (1953), Transitional objects and transitional phenomena: A study of the first not-me possession. In: *Collected Papers*. New York: Basic Books, 1958, pp. 229–242.

——— (1960a), Ego distortion in terms of true and false self. In: *The Maturational Processes and the Facilitating Environment*. New York: International Universities Press, 1965, pp. 140–152.

——— (1960b), The theory of the parent–infant relationship. In: *The Maturational Processes and the Facilitating Environment*. New York: International Universities Press, 1965, pp. 37–55.

——— (1962), Ego integration in child development. In: *The Maturational Processes and the Facilitating Environment*. New York: International Universities Press, 1965, pp. 56–63.

——— (1963a), Communicating and not communicating leading to a study of certain opposites. In: *The Maturational Processes and the Facilitating Environment*. New York: International Universities Press, 1965, pp. 179–192.

——— (1963b), Fear of breakdown. In: *Psychoanalytic Explorations*. Cambridge, MA: Harvard University Press, 1989, pp. 87–95.

———— (1963c), From dependence towards independence in the development of the individual. In: *The Maturational Processes and the Facilitating Environment*. New York: International Universities Press, 1965, pp. 83–92.

———— (1968), Psychotherapy in the designed therapeutic milieu. *Internat. Psychiatric Clinics*, 5:3–11. Boston: Little, Brown.

Name Index

Subject Index